Professional Confidence

Navigating Corporate Culture, Leadership Roles and Job Interviews

Michelle Mann

Copyright © 2023 by Michelle Mann

All rights reserved.

No portion of this book may be reproduced in any form without written permission from the publisher or author, except as permitted by U.S. copyright law.

Contents

1. Introduction — 1
2. The Evolution of Corporate Culture — 13
3. Work-life Balance in the Modern Era — 23
4. Mastering Interpersonal Relationships in the Workplace — 27
5. Nurturing and Maintaining Those Relationships — 37
6. Adapting Communication Based on Others' Needs — 45
7. Mastering Interpersonal Relationships in the Workplace — 50
8. Avoiding unconscious biases — 64
9. Branding Yourself: Your Professional Identity — 80
10. Strategies for Successful Networking Events — 92
11. Thriving in Job Interviews — 101
12. Navigating Career Changes and Transitions — 114
13. Achieving Work-Life Balance in a Demanding World — 120
14. Lifelong Learning and Continued Professional Development — 137
15. The Role of Certifications and Advanced Degrees — 153

16. Conclusion 157

Chapter One

Introduction

In the dynamic theater of professional pursuits, where the spotlight is often harsh, and the stakes are high, confidence emerges as the unsung hero—the secret ingredient that transforms competence into influence. Picture this book as your backstage pass to the grand production of your career, where the script is ever-changing, and the applause is reserved for those who command the stage with unshakeable assurance. "Professional Confidence: Navigating Corporate Culture, Leadership Roles, and Job Interviews" is more than a book; it's your invitation to step into the limelight with poise and purpose.

Confidence, at its core, is not a display of arrogance but a quiet understanding of one's capabilities. It's the steady hand that guides you through the fog of uncertainty, the unwavering voice that speaks your truth amid the cacophony of opinions. As we embark on this journey together, let's strip away the misconceptions surrounding confidence. It's not a mask to wear but a state of being to embrace—a force that emanates from authenticity, competence, and a profound belief in your capacity to make a difference.

Imagine confidence as the compass that points you north in the ever-shifting terrain of the professional world. It's not about putting on a show or projecting an image; it's about aligning your actions with your convictions, about navigating the labyrinth of challenges with a steady hand and a clear vision. In the pages that follow, we'll dissect the anatomy of this powerful force, exploring its roots, branches, and the myriad ways it intertwines with every aspect of your professional life.

The journey to professional confidence is not a sprint but a marathon—a continuous evolution marked by self-discovery and resilience. It's about understanding that setbacks are not roadblocks but stepping stones, each one refining your character and strengthening your resolve. As we delve into the nuances of confidence, I encourage you to view challenges not as threats but as opportunities for growth, as invitations to embrace discomfort and emerge on the other side, more resilient and self-assured.

This book is your companion in the quest for genuine confidence—the kind that transcends fleeting victories and withstands the tests of time. We'll explore the delicate dance between humility and assertiveness, the art of gracefully recovering from failures, and the strategies to cultivate a mindset that thrives in adversity. Confidence, in its truest form, is not a shield against vulnerability but a source of strength that arises from acknowledging and embracing your vulnerabilities.

Think of confidence as a muscle that requires regular exercise. Each chapter is designed to be a workout, challenging you to stretch beyond your comfort zone, to flex your intellectual and emotional muscles, and to build endurance in the face of uncertainty. Just as a seasoned athlete refines their skills through disciplined practice, you, too, will refine your confidence through deliberate actions and a commitment to continuous improvement.

In the grand symphony of your career, confidence is the melody that resonates across boardrooms, echoes through meetings, and leaves an indelible imprint on every interaction. It's the undercurrent that influences not only how others perceive you but, more importantly, how you perceive yourself. As we navigate the chapters ahead, remember that confidence is not a commodity to be gained or lost; it's a reservoir within you, waiting to be tapped into and shared with the world.

So, let the curtain rise on this exploration of professional confidence. With each turn of the page, envision yourself stepping onto a stage illuminated by the spotlight of your potential. The script is yours to write, and confidence is your guiding star. Embrace the journey, savor the challenges, and revel in the knowledge that you have within you the power to unleash a level of professional confidence that transcends boundaries and propels you toward unparalleled success.

The Importance of Confidence in the Corporate Landscape

Before we dive into the intricacies of professional prowess, let's ponder on a fundamental truth—the undeniable significance of confidence. Confidence isn't merely a personality trait; it's a dynamic force that shapes perceptions, opens doors, and propels you toward success. Whether you're angling for that corner office, preparing for a leadership role, or acing a crucial job interview, confidence is your silent partner, whispering courage in your ear when faced with challenges.

Let's embark on a deeper exploration of the pivotal role that confidence plays in the intricate combination of the corporate landscape. In the grand theater of professional life, confidence is the spotlight that not only highlights your skills and capabilities but also casts a transformative glow on your entire professional persona.

Consider for a moment the scenario of a boardroom presentation. The presenter who exudes confidence doesn't just share information;

they command attention. It's not about having all the answers, but about having the poise to handle the unknowns with grace. Confidence isn't an embellishment; it's the foundation upon which trust, credibility, and influence are built.

In the vast ocean of corporate interactions, from casual coffee chats to high-stakes negotiations, confidence is the sail that propels your proverbial ship. It's what separates the memorable from the forgettable, the influential from the inconspicuous. When you walk into a room with confidence, you aren't just an observer; you become an active participant in the unfolding narrative of your career.

Let's dissect this further. Confidence is not a singular trait; it's a multi-faceted gem with facets that include self-assurance, self-awareness, and a profound understanding of one's strengths and areas for growth. It's the inner compass that guides you through uncertainty and the anchor that keeps you grounded amidst success. Confidence is not an arrogant proclamation of superiority but a quiet assurance that emanates from competence and authenticity.

The corporate landscape, much like the natural world, is governed by the principles of survival of the fittest. In this context, 'fittest' doesn't necessarily mean the one with the most technical skills or the highest IQ. It's often the individual who can navigate ambiguity with confidence, adapt to change with resilience, and communicate with clarity who rises to the top.

Consider, for instance, the trajectory of a project manager entrusted with leading a diverse team through a challenging project. Beyond technical expertise, what sets apart an exemplary leader is the confidence to make decisions, take calculated risks, and inspire the team through periods of uncertainty. Confidence, in this context, becomes the glue that binds a team together, the force that transforms challenges into opportunities.

Furthermore, confidence is infectious. It creates a positive feedback loop wherein your belief in yourself inspires confidence in those around you. As a leader, your team looks to you not just for direction but for assurance. Your confidence becomes a source of motivation, a reminder that challenges are surmountable, and success is attainable.

In the realm of corporate culture, where networking is as vital as skill acquisition, confidence serves as your passport to meaningful connections. Whether you're engaging in water cooler conversations or presenting ideas in a boardroom, the ability to communicate with assurance builds bridges. It's not just about what you say; it's about how you say it. Confidence in communication is the art of expressing ideas with conviction, the skill of making your voice heard in a sea of opinions.

Moreover, confidence is a shield against the pitfalls of imposter syndrome—a phenomenon that plagues even the most accomplished professionals. It's the inner voice that says, "I belong here; I have earned my place." When faced with challenges or setbacks, confidence acts as a resilient force, allowing you to view failures not as insurmountable obstacles but as stepping stones toward growth and improvement.

To tie it together, confidence is not a luxury reserved for the chosen few; it's a prerequisite for success in the competitive arena of the professional world. It's the catalyst that transforms potential into performance and aspirations into achievements. As we navigate the chapters ahead, we'll delve deeper into the intricacies of building and sustaining this invaluable trait, understanding that confidence is not just a tool in your professional toolkit; it's the master key that unlocks the doors to your full potential.

This book delves deep into the psyche of professional confidence, unraveling its layers and unveiling the secrets to harnessing it effectively. We explore how confidence isn't a static attribute but a skill that can be honed and refined, adapting to different scenarios and stages of your career.

The Modern Man's Guide to Excelling in the Professional World

In the past, the corporate landscape might have seemed like a chessboard with a predetermined set of moves. Today, it's more akin to a dynamic game of poker, where adaptability, resilience, and, above all, confidence are the winning cards. "Professional Confidence" is crafted with the modern man in mind, someone who understands that success is not guaranteed by simply following the rules but by knowing when to bend and break them strategically.

In the dynamic pairing of the modern professional world, where change is the only constant and adaptability is a prized skill, the need for a comprehensive guide has never been more crucial. This isn't just a book; it's your passport to not just survival but triumph in a landscape that demands not only expertise but a strategic blend of charisma, adaptability, and unwavering confidence.

As we stand on the precipice of a new era in professional dynamics, the expectations and demands on the modern man have evolved. Gone are the days when success was a linear path, and climbing the corporate ladder was a predictable journey. Today, the professional journey is more like navigating a bustling metropolis—filled with opportunities, challenges, and the need for a keen sense of direction.

This book is your virtual mentor, your strategic ally in this journey through the intricate corridors of the professional realm. It's crafted with the understanding that the modern man is not defined by a rigid set of characteristics but by the ability to evolve, pivot, and thrive in an environment that is as unpredictable as it is promising.

Understanding the Modern Professional Landscape

To excel in the professional world today requires more than just technical prowess. It demands a holistic approach that encompasses emotional intelligence, adaptability, and a keen understanding of the ever-shifting currents of corporate culture. This isn't just a guide to climbing the corporate ladder; it's a manual for navigating the labyrinth of contemporary professional life.

In this context, 'modern' doesn't merely refer to a specific generation but to a mindset—a mindset that embraces change, values diversity, and recognizes the power of collaboration. The modern man is not bound by traditional notions of hierarchy but thrives in a culture that fosters innovation, inclusivity, and continuous learning.

As we embark on a profound exploration of the contemporary professional landscape, it's imperative to recognize that the terrain has evolved into a dynamic ecosystem, a harmony, woven with the threads of globalization, technological revolution, and a shifting socio-cultural fabric. The modern professional is not merely a player in this landscape; they are an adaptive strategist, a navigator who must decipher the nuanced language of success in an ever-changing environment.

Gone are the days when a linear career trajectory could be meticulously planned and adhered to without deviation. The modern professional landscape resembles more of a labyrinth than a straightforward path. The rules of engagement are not etched in stone but are rather written in the fluid ink of adaptability and innovation.

One of the defining characteristics of this new era is the dismantling of traditional career structures. The rigid hierarchies of yesteryears have given way to a more egalitarian ethos where merit, creativity, and collaboration take precedence over tenure and formal titles. The modern professional is not confined to climbing a predetermined corporate ladder; instead, they navigate a web of opportunities, lateral moves, and entrepreneurial endeavors.

Globalization, as both a challenge and an opportunity, has redefined the scope of professional interactions. The modern professional is not confined by geographical boundaries; they engage in a borderless dance of collaboration, competition, and cultural exchange. The ability to navigate this global dance floor with finesse requires a set of skills that extends beyond technical expertise—cultural intelligence, adaptability, and effective communication become the currencies that facilitate success on this international stage.

Technological integration, another hallmark of the modern professional landscape, has transformed not only the nature of work but also the skills demanded in the marketplace. Automation and artificial intelligence have become integral players in the professional orchestra, reshaping job descriptions and creating new avenues of opportunity. The modern professional is not threatened by these technological advances but rather embraces them as tools for efficiency, innovation, and creativity.

Moreover, the socio-cultural fabric of the professional world has undergone a profound metamorphosis. Diversity and inclusion are not just buzzwords but imperatives for success. The modern professional understands that a diverse team, reflective of varied perspectives and backgrounds, is a wellspring of innovation and resilience. Inclusivity is not a checkbox to be ticked but a mindset to be cultivated—a recognition that the strength of a team lies in its diversity.

Against this backdrop of complexity and change, the modern professional is akin to an agile navigator, steering through uncertainties with a compass forged from a unique blend of skills, attitudes, and a keen understanding of the larger landscape. It's not just about what you know; it's about how you adapt, collaborate, and continuously learn in the face of evolving challenges.

As we delve into the chapters ahead, it's crucial to view professional development not as a destination but as a continuous journey. The modern professional understands that stagnation is the enemy of progress and that learning is not a phase but a lifelong commitment. The ability to upskill, reskill, and embrace the dynamics of change becomes a superpower in this landscape.

Additionally, emotional intelligence emerges as a cornerstone of success in the modern professional world. The capacity to understand and navigate one's own emotions, as well as those of others, becomes a skill as essential as any technical proficiency. The ability to foster meaningful connections, lead with empathy, and navigate the delicate intricacies of human interactions distinguishes the successful modern professional from the rest.

In a nut shell, understanding the modern professional landscape is not just about recognizing external shifts; it's about cultivating an internal compass that guides you through the complexities and uncertainties. The modern professional is not a passive spectator but an active participant in shaping their own narrative, understanding that success is not a fixed point on the horizon but a journey of continuous evolution. As we unravel the layers of this dynamic landscape, let us embrace the spirit of curiosity, adaptability, and resilience, for in doing so, we equip ourselves not just for the challenges of today but for the ever-evolving landscape of tomorrow.

Adapting to the Winds of Change

The winds of change in the professional world are blowing with hurricane force. Technological advancements, global connectivity, and the evolving expectations of a diverse workforce have reshaped the landscape. The modern man is not resistant to change but embraces it as an opportunity for growth. This book serves as your compass, helping you not only navigate change but leverage it to your advantage.

We delve into the importance of adaptability as a cornerstone of success in the modern professional landscape. From embracing new technologies to navigating remote work dynamics, the chapters ahead provide insights and strategies to not just survive but thrive in an environment where the only constant is change.

Charisma Beyond Charm: The Art of Effective Communication

In an era where communication is not just about transmitting information but building meaningful connections, the modern man understands that charisma goes beyond surface charm. It's about the ability to articulate ideas with clarity, to listen actively, and to communicate authentically. This book unravels the layers of effective communication, offering practical tips and strategies to make your voice not just heard but valued in the cacophony of professional interactions.

Charisma, in the context of this guide, is not a mystical quality possessed by a select few. It's a skill that can be cultivated and refined, whether you're leading a team, negotiating a deal, or simply navigating a networking event. From body language to the art of storytelling, we explore the elements that contribute to building a magnetic presence in the professional arena.

Strategic Confidence: Beyond the Surface

While confidence is often perceived as a surface-level trait, the modern man understands that it goes beyond a mere show of bravado. Strategic confidence is about understanding your strengths, acknowledging your areas for improvement, and navigating challenges with a quiet assurance. This book takes you on a journey through the psychology of confidence, offering tools and exercises to build a reservoir of resilience that empowers you in the face of uncertainty.

Strategic confidence is not about being immune to self-doubt but about developing the tools to confront and conquer it. As we progress through the chapters, we'll explore strategies to overcome imposter syndrome, build a robust sense of self-belief, and project an aura of confidence that is both authentic and impactful.

Tailoring Success: Your Unique Professional Journey

The modern man's journey to success is not a one-size-fits-all narrative. This book acknowledges and celebrates the uniqueness of your path. Whether you're charting a course in a traditional corporate setting, navigating the entrepreneurial landscape, or exploring the gig economy, the principles and strategies presented here are adaptable to your individual circumstances.

Success, in the context of this guide, is not a destination but a continuous journey of growth and self-discovery. It's about setting and achieving meaningful goals, cultivating a fulfilling professional life, and finding a harmonious balance between ambition and well-being. Each chapter provides insights and tools to tailor success to your unique aspirations and circumstances.

As we journey through the pages of this guide, envision it not just as a source of information but as a dynamic companion on your professional odyssey. Consider it your co-pilot, offering guidance, inspiration, and practical strategies to navigate the twists and turns of the modern professional landscape. The destination? A future where success is not just a goal but a way of life, and the modern man is not just a participant but a trailblazer in the ever-evolving saga of professional excellence.

This book isn't a one-size-fits-all manual. It's a personalized guide, acknowledging the uniqueness of your journey and offering insights that can be tailored to your individual circumstances. From the entry-level professional seeking to make a mark to the seasoned executive aiming for the C-suite, the principles explored here are versatile, adaptable, and applicable to professionals at every stage of their career.

What Readers Can Expect and How to Best Utilize the Book

Consider this book as your arsenal, packed with practical strategies, real-world anecdotes, and actionable advice. Each chapter is a tool designed to sharpen a specific aspect of your professional persona. Whether you're struggling with imposter syndrome, seeking ways to communicate with authority, or looking for the secrets to acing interviews, there's a dedicated section to guide you.

The chapters are structured to provide not just knowledge but a roadmap for application. You'll find exercises, reflection points, and tangible action steps that transform theoretical concepts into practical habits. This isn't a book you read and put on the shelf; it's a resource you return to, a mentor you consult as you navigate the twists and turns of your career.

As you embark on this journey through the pages of "Professional Confidence," I encourage you to approach it with an open mind and a willingness to challenge yourself. Confidence, after all, is not a spectator sport. It demands participation, engagement, and a commitment to growth. Consider this book your ally in that pursuit.

In the chapters that follow, we'll explore the foundations of confidence, the nuances of effective communication, the art of leadership, and the strategies to master the daunting realm of job interviews. Together, we'll unravel the mysteries of the professional world, armed with the unwavering belief that confidence is not a luxury; it's a necessity.

So, fasten your seatbelt, dear reader. The journey to professional excellence begins now, and your destination is a future where confidence isn't just a trait; it's a way of life.

Chapter Two

The Evolution of Corporate Culture

In the grand masterpieces of professional success, the thread that weaves through every achievement, every milestone, and every innovation is corporate culture. It's the silent force that shapes the identity of an organization, influencing not just its internal dynamics but also its standing in the marketplace. As we embark on this exploration of the evolution of corporate culture, we peel back the layers of history to understand how it has transformed from a mere backdrop to a strategic cornerstone of success.

The journey begins not in the boardrooms of contemporary skyscrapers but in the industrial landscapes of the early 20th century. The inception of corporate culture can be traced back to an era where factories hummed with productivity, and the organizational structure mirrored the assembly lines that defined the manufacturing age. It was a time when efficiency was the heartbeat of corporate philosophy, and the workplace was characterized by a top-down approach where directives trickled from the executive suite to the factory floor.

However, as industries burgeoned and the workforce diversified, a subtle shift began to ripple through the organizational fabric. The realization dawned that success wasn't solely dependent on mechanical efficiency but on the human element—on the engagement, satisfaction, and collaboration of the workforce. This marked the birth of a more inclusive corporate culture, one that acknowledged the importance of employee morale and well-being.

Fast forward to the latter half of the 20th century, and the landscape of corporate culture underwent a seismic shift. The rigid hierarchies of the past began to crumble, making way for a more egalitarian approach. The workplace was no longer a battleground of authority but a collaborative space where ideas could flourish irrespective of rank or title. This era saw the emergence of values-driven cultures, where companies sought to define and live by a set of principles that extended beyond profit margins.

The Silicon Valley boom of the late 20th century further accelerated the evolution of corporate culture. Tech giants like Apple and Google became synonymous not only with innovation but also with vibrant, employee-centric cultures. The notion that a positive workplace culture could be a competitive advantage gained traction, leading to a paradigm shift where the employee experience was prioritized as a driver of success.

In the 21st century, corporate culture has become a buzzword, but its essence goes beyond mere rhetoric. It's not about ping pong tables and free snacks; it's about creating an environment where individuals feel valued, empowered, and inspired to contribute their best. The evolution continues, shaped by the digital age, the gig economy, and a globalized workforce.

Today, corporate culture is a strategic imperative. Organizations recognize that attracting and retaining top talent is not just about salaries and benefits but about fostering an environment where employees thrive. The culture is no longer a byproduct but a deliberate creation—a delicate ecosystem where innovation, diversity, and inclusion flourish.

As we traverse the pages of this chapter, we'll delve into the key milestones that have marked the evolution of corporate culture. From the era of industrial efficiency to the age of innovation, each phase has left its imprint on the way we perceive and cultivate workplace dynamics. We'll explore the role of leadership in shaping culture, the impact of technological advancements, and the imperative of aligning corporate values with the aspirations of the workforce.

Join me on this journey through time and change as we unravel the layers of corporate culture, understanding not just where it has been but where it is headed. As Doug Conant wisely asserted, winning in the marketplace is intricately linked to winning in the workplace. Let's explore how the evolution of corporate culture is not just a historical narrative but a roadmap to success in the ever-evolving landscape of the professional world.

Understanding Historical Context

To comprehend the evolution of corporate culture, we must first dissect the historical roots that anchored the traditional corporate ladder—a structure that once defined professional ascent. Picture a landscape where success was symbolized by a linear climb, where each step on the hierarchical ladder brought one closer to the pinnacle of corporate achievement.

The traditional corporate ladder, while an established symbol of progress, came with its inherent limitations. It often promoted a siloed approach, where individuals operated within their designated spheres, seldom engaging with colleagues beyond their immediate teams. This structure, while providing a clear trajectory for career advancement, inadvertently stifled the free flow of ideas and collaboration.

The turning point in this historical narrative came with a realization—the recognition that organizational success was not solely predicated on individual achievement but on the collective strength of a diverse and collaborative workforce. Hence, the rigid rungs of the traditional ladder began to give way to a more flexible, adaptive structure that encouraged lateral movement and cross-functional collaboration.

The shift towards flexible structures was not a mere organizational facelift but a profound reimagining of the workplace ecosystem. In this contemporary landscape, success was no longer measured solely by vertical ascension but also by the ability to navigate laterally, to explore diverse roles and perspectives. The flexible structure became a reflection of an organization's adaptability—a crucial trait in a rapidly changing business environment.

Collaboration emerged as a central theme in this evolution. The insular climb of the traditional ladder gave way to a collective journey where teams collaborated across departments and hierarchies. This marked a departure from the top-down communication style to a more inclusive, participative approach. The synergy of diverse minds working together became the catalyst for innovation and problem-solving.

Diversity, as a driving force, played a pivotal role in reshaping corporate dynamics. Organizations came to understand that a homogenous workforce stifles creativity and limits adaptability. The emphasis shifted from viewing diversity as a compliance requirement to recognizing it as a strategic advantage. Inclusivity became the mantra, creating environments where individuals felt empowered to bring their authentic selves to the workplace.

However, the historical context of the corporate ladder's evolution signifies more than a chronological progression—it represents a fundamental shift in mindset. It's a transition from a linear, individual-centric model to a dynamic, collaborative ecosystem. Join me as we delve deeper into the intricacies of this transformation, uncovering the motivations and implications that have shaped the corporate culture we navigate today.

Modern Corporate Values and Expectations

In the kaleidoscopic landscape of modern corporate culture, a new chapter is unfolding—one marked by a redefinition of values and a recalibration of expectations. As organizations strive for relevance in an era of rapid change, they are compelled to weave ethical considerations, social responsibility, and a nuanced understanding of the human element into the very fabric of their identity.

Ethical Considerations and Social Responsibility:

In the tapestry of modern corporate values, ethical considerations and social responsibility form the vibrant threads that not only color an organization's character but also shape its legacy. Gone are the days when corporate ethics was confined to boardroom discussions; it has emerged as a guiding philosophy, a moral compass that directs the course of decision-making.

In the relentless pursuit of profit, organizations now acknowledge a dual responsibility—to their stakeholders and the global community. The ethical considerations go beyond mere compliance; they delve into the intricacies of fair labor practices, environmental sustainability, and the impact of operations on local communities.

Moreover, social responsibility has evolved from a philanthropic gesture to an integral part of a company's identity. Whether it's championing social causes, promoting diversity and inclusion, or engaging in initiatives that uplift communities, organizations are recognizing their role as catalysts for positive change. We explore the strategies employed by corporations to embed social responsibility into their DNA, creating a ripple effect that extends far beyond the confines of their offices.

As we navigate through this terrain, it becomes evident that ethical considerations and social responsibility are not mere checkboxes on a corporate agenda. They are the narrative arc that defines the character of organizations, distinguishing those that merely exist from those that leave an indelible mark on the world. Join me as we unravel the narratives of ethical pioneers and socially responsible trailblazers, understanding how these principles are shaping the very jist of modern corporate culture.

The Rise of Remote Work and Its Implications

The seismic tremors of change reverberate in the traditional understanding of work as we witness the meteoric rise of remote work. Accelerated by global circumstances and empowered by technological advances, remote work is not just a temporary disruption but a paradigm shift. This section navigates the uncharted waters of this revolution, exploring its implications on corporate culture. How does one foster a sense of belonging and shared purpose when teams are scattered across geographical distances? What leadership styles thrive in a virtual realm? We embark on a journey into the digital frontier, uncovering the strategies employed by organizations to adapt and thrive in this new reality.

In traversing the realms of modern corporate values and expectations, we discover a narrative that extends beyond profit and loss statements. It's a narrative of conscious capitalism, where success is not just measured by financial gains but by the positive imprint an organization leaves on society. Join me as we explore this dynamic landscape, where ethics, soft skills, and the remote work revolution converge to redefine the very essence of what it means to be successful in the modern corporate world.

In the grand tapestry of professional fulfillment, the alignment of personal values with corporate culture emerges as a nuanced dance—one that requires self-awareness, deliberate choices, and the orchestration of a harmonious partnership between individual aspirations and organizational ethos.

The overture to this dance is self-reflection—a journey into the inner sanctum of one's beliefs and priorities. It's a process that demands time, introspection, and an honest appraisal of what truly matters. In a world often characterized by the hustle and bustle of daily tasks, this chapter encourages professionals to pause and engage in a profound dialogue with themselves. What are the core values that define success for you? What are the non-negotiables that shape your professional identity? Self-reflection becomes the compass that points toward authenticity—a guiding force in navigating the intricate terrain of corporate culture.

As individuals embark on this introspective journey, the role of corporate missions and visions emerges as a guiding star. A well-crafted mission statement transcends the realm of mere rhetoric; it becomes a declaration of purpose—a shared vision that beckons like-minded individuals. This section explores how aligning personal values with an organization's mission creates a magnetic force, attracting individuals who not only contribute to the workplace but find profound meaning in doing so. We delve into case studies, exploring organizations where the marriage of individual purpose with corporate vision propels both the employee and the company toward unprecedented heights.

However, as in any dance, not every step is seamless. The spotlight then shifts to the challenges of navigating value mismatches. In a world of diverse organizations, each with its unique culture, individuals may find themselves in environments that don't perfectly align with their values. This chapter provides a roadmap for professionals facing such disparities, addressing the complexities of compromise, negotiation, and, in some cases, the courageous decision to seek a more congruent partnership elsewhere.

Moreover, we explore the dynamic nature of personal values and corporate culture. The dance isn't a one-time performance but an ongoing collaboration that evolves with the individual and the organization. Strategies for staying attuned to these changes, for recalibrating when necessary, and fostering a workplace that embraces growth and transformation are integral components of this exploration.

Impact of Tech and Innovation on Culture

In the ever-evolving saga of the modern workplace, the profound impact of technology and innovation on corporate culture is a narrative that unfolds with each technological leap.

The first movement in this symphony of change is the evolution of communication tools—a historical progression that mirrors the evolution of societal connectivity. From the days of memos and interoffice mail to the instantaneous, interconnected realm of digital platforms, the medium through which teams communicate has undergone a seismic shift. This exploration not only traces the trajectory of communication tools but delves into their transformative influence on workplace dynamics. The speed of communication is not just a logistical shift; it is a fundamental transformation in how teams connect, collaborate, and cultivate a shared sense of purpose. Case studies illuminate the ways in which this evolution has reshaped organizational hierarchies, flattened communication structures, and fostered a culture of inclusivity and immediacy.

A pivotal note in this exploration is the rise of digital-first strategies. Organizations no longer view technology as a mere tool but as a strategic ally in shaping and defining culture. We navigate through the corridors of digital transformation, dissecting how embracing digital platforms for collaboration, project management, and communication can foster an environment of agility and responsiveness. Real-world examples highlight the profound impact of these strategies on the adaptability and resilience of organizational cultures, showcasing instances where technology becomes not just an enabler but a cultural cornerstone.

Yet, as technology takes center stage, the question of balance becomes crucial. The narrative pivots to the delicate art of balancing tech skills with the human touch. In an era where algorithms and artificial intelligence play integral roles, the human element remains irreplaceable. This chapter unfolds as a thoughtful exploration of how organizations navigate the fine line between automation and maintaining a workplace culture that values empathy, creativity, and authentic human connections. Interviews with industry leaders shed light on how successful organizations leverage technology without sacrificing the essence of human-centric cultures, emphasizing that even in the age of algorithms, it is the human touch that distinguishes thriving workplaces.

Moreover, staying updated in the ever-accelerating tech landscape becomes a mandate for professionals navigating this digital frontier. The chapter expands on strategies for continuous learning and adaptation, acknowledging that in a world of rapid technological evolution, standing still is akin to stepping backward. Through practical insights, we equip professionals not only to cope with technological shifts but to thrive amidst them, transforming challenges into opportunities for personal and organizational growth.

Chapter Three

Work-life Balance in the Modern Era

In the dynamic landscape of the modern workplace, achieving a harmonious work-life balance has become a pursuit of paramount importance. The first brushstroke on this canvas explores the changing boundaries of work and home—a transformation accelerated by the advent of remote work and digital connectivity. The traditional nine-to-five paradigm has given way to a more fluid, interconnected existence where the office is not a place but a state of mind. We examine the benefits and challenges of this paradigm shift, understanding how professionals navigate the blurred lines between work and personal life. Real-world anecdotes shed light on innovative approaches to achieving balance in an era where the distinction between the professional and the personal is increasingly nuanced.

A poignant movement in this exploration is the role of mental health in corporate culture. The modern workplace is not merely a venue for task completion; it is a space where mental well-being plays a pivotal role in individual and collective success. We delve into the initiatives taken by forward-thinking organizations to prioritize mental health, understanding that a healthy workforce is not just a moral imperative but a strategic advantage. Interviews with mental health experts provide insights into creating cultures that destigmatize mental health challenges and foster environments where individuals can thrive holistically.

The narrative then unfolds to the strategic art of setting boundaries for personal well-being—a skill that has become indispensable in the age of constant connectivity. We explore practical strategies for professionals to establish clear boundaries, safeguard their personal time, and nurture their mental and emotional well-being. Case studies illuminate instances where organizations actively support employees in boundary-setting, recognizing that a workforce that feels respected and valued is not only more productive but also more loyal and engaged.

In the corporate culture, the role of mental health has transcended the realm of peripheral concern to become a central tenet that defines the success and well-being of both individuals and organizations. As we delve deeper into this crucial aspect, we uncover the layers of understanding, destigmatization, and active cultivation of mental well-being within the fabric of corporate culture.

The workplace, once perceived primarily as a venue for professional tasks, has evolved into a space where mental health is not only acknowledged but actively prioritized. Mental well-being is now recognized as a cornerstone of individual and collective success. The transformation is not merely a reflection of societal shifts but a strategic imperative—an acknowledgment that a healthy, thriving workforce is a competitive advantage.

One pivotal note in this symphony is the destigmatization of mental health challenges. Traditionally, discussions around mental health were often shrouded in silence and shame. However, the narrative is changing. Forward-thinking organizations are fostering environments where open conversations about mental health are not just encouraged but embraced. The goal is not to create a facade of perfection but to acknowledge the multifaceted nature of individuals, recognizing that mental health is as vital as physical health.

Mental health initiatives within corporate culture encompass a spectrum of strategies. From employee assistance programs providing confidential counseling services to mindfulness and stress reduction workshops, organizations are proactively addressing the well-being of their workforce. This isn't merely a checklist of benefits; it's a commitment to creating a workplace where individuals feel seen, heard, and supported in their holistic development.

Moreover, mental health is no longer viewed in isolation but as part of a broader ecosystem that includes emotional, social, and even spiritual well-being. The understanding has shifted from reacting to mental health crises to proactively creating an environment that fosters psychological resilience. Training programs that equip leaders with the skills to recognize and respond to signs of mental distress are becoming integral components of organizational strategies.

In interviews with mental health experts, we gain insights into the importance of organizational culture in shaping mental well-being. The emphasis is not just on intervention but on prevention—an understanding that a workplace that actively supports mental health is one where individuals are less likely to experience burnout, disengagement, or other mental health challenges.

The significance of mental health in corporate culture extends beyond individual well-being to organizational performance. Studies consistently demonstrate that workplaces with a positive approach to mental health experience higher levels of employee engagement, productivity, and retention. The correlation is not coincidental but a testament to the interconnectedness of employee well-being and organizational success.

As we navigate the intricate terrain of mental health in corporate culture, the narrative is not one of prescription but empowerment. It's about equipping organizations with the knowledge and tools to create environments where mental health is not a marginalized concern but an integral aspect of thriving. The goal is not perfection but progress—an ongoing commitment to learning, adapting, and fostering cultures where individuals are not merely cogs in a machine but valued contributors to a collective success story.

Chapter Four

Mastering Interpersonal Relationships in the Workplace

In the professional world, where success is not only about what you know but also about who you know, mastering interpersonal relationships emerges as a skill of paramount importance. This chapter is your guide to navigating the delicate nuances of workplace connections, fostering meaningful collaborations, and building a network that extends beyond mere professional acquaintanceship.

Before we dive into the art of mastering interpersonal relationships, it's essential to understand the intricate dynamics that shape these connections. The workplace is a microcosm of personalities, ambitions, and diverse perspectives. Navigating this terrain requires not just technical expertise but a high degree of emotional intelligence—the ability to understand, empathize, and communicate effectively with colleagues at all levels.

In this section, we'll explore the different types of workplace relationships, from hierarchical connections with supervisors and subordinates to lateral collaborations with peers. Each type demands a unique set of interpersonal skills, and understanding these dynamics lays the foundation for building relationships that contribute to both personal and professional growth.

At the heart of every meaningful relationship lies empathy. This is not just a buzzword but a potent force that bridges gaps, fosters understanding, and creates a positive work environment. We'll delve into the ways you can cultivate and express empathy in the workplace, from active listening techniques to putting yourself in others' shoes. As you master the art of empathy, you'll find that it not only enhances your interpersonal relationships but also contributes to a collaborative and harmonious workplace culture.

Communication is the lifeblood of workplace relationships. In this section, we'll explore the nuances of effective communication—how to convey your ideas clearly, articulate your thoughts with confidence, and, equally importantly, listen actively. From mastering the art of constructive feedback to navigating challenging conversations, this chapter equips you with the tools to communicate with impact and finesse.

Your professional network is more than just a list of contacts; it's a strategic asset that can open doors to opportunities, mentorship, and career advancement. In this part of the chapter, we'll explore the principles of networking, both within and outside your organization. From cultivating genuine connections to leveraging social platforms, you'll learn how to build a robust professional network that serves as a valuable resource throughout your career.

Conflicts are inevitable in any workplace, but how you navigate them can make the difference between strained relationships and constructive resolutions. This section delves into conflict resolution strategies, emphasizing the importance of addressing conflicts promptly, maintaining professionalism, and finding common ground. By mastering the art of conflict resolution, you'll transform workplace challenges into opportunities for growth and strengthened relationships.

The most successful professionals understand the significance of contributing to a positive and inclusive work environment. In this final section, we'll explore how your actions and attitudes contribute to the overall workplace culture. From fostering inclusivity to celebrating diversity, you'll discover how creating a positive environment not only enhances your relationships but also elevates the collective success of your team and organization.

As we journey through this chapter, remember that mastering interpersonal relationships is not a one-time achievement but an ongoing process of learning, adapting, and growing. Your ability to connect with others, communicate effectively, and contribute to a positive work culture will not only define your professional success but also enrich the overall tapestry of your career. So, let's embark on this exploration of mastering interpersonal relationships, knowing that the skills you cultivate here will serve as pillars of strength in your professional journey.

Building Trust and Rapport

In the intricate web of workplace relationships, trust is the glue that binds. Here, we explore the art of cultivating trust and rapport, understanding that the foundation of any meaningful professional connection is built on authenticity, consistency, and open communication.

First Impressions and Their Lasting Impact:

When it comes to professional relationships, the spotlight often falls on the opening act—your first impression. It's a moment of silent communication, a dance of body language, tone, and unspoken cues that set the stage for the narrative of your relationship with a colleague. Understanding the intricacies of first impressions is not just a matter of courtesy; it's a strategic endeavor with far-reaching consequences.

The significance of a first impression lies in its permanence. Research suggests that it takes mere seconds for someone to form an initial judgment, and once formed, these impressions tend to persist over time. This phenomenon, known as the "halo effect," influences how others perceive your competence, trustworthiness, and overall suitability as a colleague.

Consider the scenario of entering a conference room for a meeting with a new team. Your posture, facial expressions, and how you articulate your greetings all contribute to the immediate impression you leave. It's not about donning a mask of artificial congeniality but about projecting authenticity and confidence.

Body language, often more powerful than spoken words, becomes the canvas upon which your first impression is painted. A firm handshake, direct eye contact, and a genuine smile convey openness and confidence. Conversely, slouched shoulders, averted gaze, or fidgeting may inadvertently communicate uncertainty or disinterest.

Moreover, the tone and pitch of your voice play a crucial role in shaping first impressions. A

As you navigate the intricacies of crafting a lasting first impression, consider the context and the individuals involved. Tailor your approach based on cultural norms, industry expectations, and the unique dynamics of your workplace. Flexibility in your interactions demonstrates adaptability, a quality highly valued in dynamic professional environments.

So, as you step onto the stage of professional interactions, remember that you are the author of your narrative. Craft a first impression that reflects not just your competence but your authenticity, leaving an indelible mark that resonates long after the curtain falls on that initial encounter.

Conflict Resolution Techniques

In the dynamic landscape of the corporate world, conflict is an inevitable companion on the journey to success. However, it's not the presence of conflict that defines a workplace but rather how conflicts are managed and resolved. Conflict resolution techniques in the corporate realm are akin to a delicate dance—orchestrating a harmonious balance between differing perspectives and competing interests.

Effective conflict resolution begins with a meticulous examination of the root causes. This involves a nuanced understanding of the motivations, expectations, and underlying issues at play. Identifying these factors lays the groundwork for targeted and sustainable solutions.

Communication stands as the cornerstone of conflict resolution in the corporate context. It's not merely about the exchange of words but the art of active listening and empathetic engagement. Effective communicators during disagreements foster an environment where diverse opinions are not perceived as threats but rather as valuable contributors to the organization's growth.

Moreover, recognizing the threshold where internal resolution mechanisms may fall short is crucial. Seeking third-party mediation becomes a strategic move in situations where conflicts reach an impasse, ensuring an unbiased perspective and facilitating a resolution that aligns with organizational values. In the corporate world, mastering conflict resolution is not just a skill; it's a strategic imperative that transforms challenges into opportunities for organizational resilience and sustained success.

Identifying the Root Causes of Conflicts:

Conflict resolution begins with a deep understanding of the underlying causes. We delve into the intricacies of identifying the root causes of conflicts, emphasizing the importance of active listening and empathetic understanding. By uncovering the true sources of disagreement, you lay the groundwork for targeted and effective resolution.

Effective identification of root causes involves an empathetic approach—one that acknowledges the diverse experiences and perspectives of those involved. It requires setting aside preconceived notions and creating a safe space for open dialogue. In doing so, you not only address the immediate conflict but also lay the groundwork for preventing future misunderstandings. Ultimately, the skill of identifying root causes transforms conflict resolution from a mere Band-Aid solution to a strategic and sustainable process of healing and growth within the professional landscape.

Effective Communication During Disagreements

Disagreements in the workplace are not a sign of dysfunction; they are a natural consequence of diverse perspectives colliding. The key to transforming these moments from potential roadblocks to avenues of growth lies in effective communication.

At the heart of communication during disagreements is the art of active listening. It's not just about waiting for your turn to speak but genuinely understanding the nuances of others' viewpoints. Acknowledging differing opinions with respect and openness fosters an environment where individuals feel heard and valued.

Expressing your own viewpoint requires finesse. It involves articulating your thoughts clearly, using assertive rather than aggressive language, and avoiding personal attacks. The goal is not to prove someone wrong but to find common ground, a shared understanding that transcends individual perspectives.

Non-verbal communication also plays a significant role. Maintaining open body language, making eye contact, and moderating your tone contribute to a positive and collaborative atmosphere. These subtle cues reinforce the message that you are engaged in a constructive dialogue, not a confrontational argument.

Moreover, effective communication during disagreements involves seeking clarity. If a point is unclear, asking questions for clarification demonstrates a genuine interest in understanding the other person's perspective. This not only resolves immediate conflicts but strengthens the foundation for future positive interactions.

Seeking Third-Party Mediation When Needed

Sometimes, conflicts reach an impasse where external intervention becomes necessary. Here, we discuss the importance of recognizing when to seek third-party mediation. Whether it's a supervisor, a human resources professional, or an external mediator, involving a neutral party can provide fresh insights and facilitate a resolution that is fair and unbiased.

Conflict resolution is not just about smoothing over disagreements; it's about transforming conflicts into opportunities for growth. By mastering these techniques, you'll not only navigate the challenges of workplace conflicts with grace but also contribute to a culture of open communication and collaboration within your professional community.

Recognizing the need for external intervention is not a sign of weakness but a testament to your commitment to fair and just outcomes. A neutral third party, be it a supervisor, a human resources professional, or an external mediator, brings a fresh perspective unburdened by personal biases. Their role is not to dictate solutions but to facilitate a dialogue that leads to a resolution acceptable to all parties involved.

Third-party mediation is akin to introducing a skilled navigator into turbulent waters. They bring an objective lens, ensuring that emotions do not cloud the path to resolution. By creating a structured and impartial space for dialogue, a mediator fosters an environment where grievances can be aired, and solutions can be explored without the fear of favoritism.

Leveraging Mentorships and Alliances

In the vast landscape of professional growth, mentorships and alliances stand out as formidable tools for advancement. This section explores the strategic art of leveraging these connections—how to seek out mentors, establish meaningful relationships, and build a network that extends beyond the confines of your current professional domain.

Mentorships play a pivotal role as guiding lights in the corporate realm. Seeking out mentors is not a sign of weakness but a testament to one's commitment to growth. A mentor, often an experienced and seasoned professional, provides insights, wisdom, and a roadmap based on their own journey. In the corporate labyrinth, where decisions carry weight and trajectories are shaped by experience, a mentor becomes a trusted advisor, offering perspectives that extend beyond the confines of textbooks or formal training.

Building formal relationships with mentors is a strategic move that pays dividends throughout one's career. These relationships extend beyond casual advice; they become a source of tailored guidance, helping individuals navigate complex challenges and make informed decisions. The mentor-mentee dynamic, when nurtured with care and authenticity, creates a symbiotic exchange of knowledge and experience.

Nurturing and maintaining mentorship relationships is akin to tending to a garden. Regular communication, a genuine willingness to learn, and the ability to apply mentorship insights to real-world scenarios are essential. These relationships are not static; they evolve and deepen over time, contributing to the mentee's professional acumen and the mentor's sense of fulfillment.

Beyond mentorships, alliances play a crucial role in the corporate tapestry. Building a network within and outside the organization is an art that goes beyond casual interactions. It involves cultivating meaningful connections with colleagues, superiors, and professionals in related fields. A diverse network becomes a source of diverse perspectives, collaboration opportunities, and a safety net of support during challenging times.

In the corporate world, where the terrain is competitive and the challenges multifaceted, leveraging mentorships and alliances is not just a professional nicety; it is a strategic imperative. It's a recognition that success is often a collective achievement, and the strength of one's professional network can be a determining factor in the trajectory of one's career. These connections, carefully cultivated and strategically leveraged, become the pillars of resilience, growth, and sustained success in the ever-evolving corporate landscape.

Seeking Out Mentors and Establishing Formal Relationships:

Mentorship is a dynamic force that propels your career forward. We delve into the nuances of identifying suitable mentors, understanding how to approach them, and establishing formal relationships that are built on trust and mutual respect. Mentorship isn't just about guidance; it's about creating a symbiotic relationship where both mentor and mentee contribute to each other's growth.

Identifying suitable mentors requires a keen understanding of your own goals and aspirations. A mentor isn't just someone with impressive credentials; they are individuals whose journey aligns with your aspirations and whose insights can offer valuable guidance. Whether within or outside your organization, mentors can be found in various professional spheres. The key lies in being proactive—actively seeking individuals whose experiences resonate with your own ambitions.

Approaching potential mentors is a delicate dance of professionalism and authenticity. It involves not only expressing your admiration for their work but also articulating your own goals and aspirations. Recognizing that mentorship is a two-way street, consider how your unique skills and perspectives could contribute to the mentorship dynamic. This isn't a transactional relationship; it's a mutual exchange of knowledge and support.

Establishing formal mentorship relationships is a commitment to structured growth. This involves defining the parameters of the mentorship, clarifying expectations, and establishing a cadence for interactions. Formalizing the relationship adds a layer of accountability, ensuring that both mentor and mentee are invested in the journey.

Chapter Five

Nurturing and Maintaining Those Relationships

Building a mentorship is akin to tending to a flourishing garden. We discuss the importance of nurturing and maintaining these relationships over time. Effective communication, a willingness to learn, and a genuine appreciation for your mentor's insights contribute to a mentorship that stands the test of time. Additionally, we explore strategies for expressing gratitude and reciprocating value within the mentorship dynamic.

Building a mentorship is not a one-time endeavor; it's an ongoing cultivation of a relationship that holds the potential for a profound impact on your professional journey. The art of nurturing and maintaining these connections is akin to tending to a garden—requiring attention, care, and a genuine appreciation for the growth that ensues.

Effective communication lies at the heart of maintaining mentorship relationships. Regular check-ins, updates on your progress, and a willingness to share both challenges and triumphs create a dynamic dialogue that sustains the connection. It's not merely about seeking advice; it's about fostering a reciprocal relationship where both mentor and mentee contribute to each other's growth.

Expressing gratitude is a cornerstone of maintaining a mentorship. Acknowledging the time, insights, and guidance bestowed by your mentor reinforces the value of the relationship. Gratitude is not just a sentiment; it's a currency that strengthens the bonds of mentorship, creating an atmosphere of mutual respect and appreciation.

Reciprocity is another key element in the nurturing process. While mentors provide guidance, mentees bring fresh perspectives and enthusiasm. A mentee's success is a testament to the mentor's impact, creating a cycle of shared accomplishments. Actively seeking opportunities to reciprocate value—whether through sharing insights, offering assistance, or contributing to your mentor's projects—transforms the mentorship into a collaborative alliance.

Moreover, staying open to learning is crucial for the longevity of a mentorship. As your career evolves, so do the challenges and opportunities you encounter. A willingness to remain a perpetual learner, coupled with a receptiveness to your mentor's evolving insights, ensures that the relationship remains dynamic and relevant.

Building a Network Within and Outside the Organization

Alliances extend beyond mentorships to encompass a broader network. Here, we explore the art of building a network within and outside the organization. From cultivating relationships with colleagues and superiors to extending your reach to professionals in related fields, a diverse network becomes a source of knowledge, opportunities, and support. We discuss strategies for effective networking, both in-person and through digital platforms, that elevate your professional presence.

In the dynamic realm of professional success, the ability to build and nurture a network is akin to having a compass that points towards endless opportunities. This section unravels the art of building a network, both within the confines of your organization and beyond its borders, exploring the transformative power of strategic connections.

Within the familiar walls of your organization lies a treasure trove of connections waiting to be cultivated. Building a network within the organization involves more than casual conversations at the coffee machine—it's about intentional relationship-building. Engaging with colleagues from different departments, attending company events, and participating in cross-functional projects are avenues to weave a web of relationships that extend beyond your immediate team. These connections not only enrich your understanding of internal dynamics but also pave the way for collaborative ventures and unexpected opportunities.

The horizons of professional growth extend far beyond the boundaries of your workplace. Actively building a network outside the organization broadens your perspective, exposes you to diverse insights, and opens doors to opportunities beyond your current role. Professional associations, industry conferences, and online platforms become fertile grounds for connecting with professionals who bring a fresh lens to your field. By extending your network to individuals outside your immediate professional sphere, you create a reservoir of knowledge, mentorship, and potential collaborations that transcend organizational limitations.

Effective networking is a deliberate endeavor that requires both finesse and authenticity. It's not about collecting business cards but about forging genuine connections. We discuss strategies for effective networking, from the art of introducing yourself with impact to maintaining a consistent online presence. Leveraging social media platforms, attending industry events, and participating in professional groups are avenues to amplify your network-building efforts.

Understanding Office Politics

In the unique ecosystem of the workplace, the undercurrents of office politics flow beneath the surface, shaping dynamics and influencing professional trajectories. This section delves into the nuanced art of understanding office politics—how to recognize political landscapes, navigate power dynamics, and employ strategies that ensure success without compromising integrity.

In the workplace, imagine a big puzzle. Different pieces represent different roles, and each piece has its own importance. Office politics is about recognizing who holds what piece and understanding how decisions are made. Some people may have more influence, like the key players in a game. It's not about who's the boss; it's about understanding the different roles and how they interact.

In the workplace, you might come across situations where people try to influence decisions or form groups. Navigating office politics is like finding your way through these situations without giving up on what you believe is right. It's about staying true to yourself, making ethical choices, and deciding when to stand firm and when to find common ground with others.

Think of unnecessary drama like waves in the river that can make the journey bumpy. Navigating office politics involves strategies to avoid getting caught up in drama. It's about staying focused on your work, not getting involved in gossip, and keeping a professional attitude. By doing this, you create a smoother path for yourself and contribute to a positive work environment.

Understanding office politics doesn't mean playing games or being sneaky. It's about being aware of how things work, making smart choices, and creating a workplace where everyone can succeed while staying true to their values. So, think of it as learning to read the currents of the workplace river and steering your boat wisely to reach your professional destination smoothly.

Recognizing Political Landscapes and Power Dynamics

Office politics often mirrors the currents of a complex river, with power dynamics shaping the direction of flow. We explore the art of recognizing political landscapes, understanding hierarchies, and identifying key influencers within your organization. By deciphering the unspoken rules of power, you gain insight into how decisions are made, alliances are formed, and influence is wielded.

Imagine your workplace is a map, and on that map, some people have more influence than others. These are the political landscapes. It's about understanding who has the power and where things get decided. It's not about playing games but understanding how things work.

Now, let's talk about power dynamics. In any group, some people's words carry more weight. They might be managers or team leads, or just the go-to person. Understanding power dynamics is recognizing who can help you get things done. It's not about challenging authority but knowing how influence is spread.

Think of it like navigating a river. By recognizing political landscapes and understanding power dynamics, you get a compass. You know where the currents are strong, where there might be challenges, and where it's smooth sailing. It's not about playing politics for personal gain but using this knowledge to navigate your work environment effectively.

So, as you navigate this river of office politics, think of it as a strategic journey. By understanding the lay of the land and recognizing where the currents of influence flow, you can ensure that your boat sails smoothly

Empathy and Emotional Intelligence

In the tapestry of workplace dynamics, empathy, and emotional intelligence emerge as threads that weave connections, fostering a culture of understanding and collaboration. This section delves into the profound impact of recognizing and embracing emotions in the workplace, adapting communication to meet the needs of others, and understanding the strength found in vulnerability.

In the vibrant tapestry of the workplace, emotions weave intricate patterns, influencing the daily narrative. Here, empathy and emotional intelligence transcend abstract concepts, becoming tangible tools that foster understanding among colleagues.

Amidst the deadlines and meetings, emotions are not intruders but participants in the professional journey. Recognizing and validating emotions is an acknowledgment that each person's experience is unique. It establishes a culture where expressing feelings is not a sign of weakness but a testament to authenticity and emotional well-being.

Communication, the lifeblood of collaboration, is not a one-size-fits-all endeavor. Emotional intelligence guides us to adapt communication based on the needs of those around us. It goes beyond words, tuning into non-verbal cues—deciphering the unspoken language of body language and tone. This adaptability creates an environment where colleagues feel seen, heard, and valued, laying a crucial foundation for positive workplace relationships.

In the realm of emotional intelligence, vulnerability emerges as a profound strength. It is the courage to be open about challenges, uncertainties, and even mistakes. Far from a sign of fragility, this transparency fosters trust and authentic connections. In embracing vulnerability, the workplace transforms into a space for shared growth and resilience.

Empathy and emotional intelligence are not mere workplace buzzwords; they are keys to unlocking a culture of understanding, compassion, and collective success. By recognizing and validating emotions, adapting communication, and embracing vulnerability, you contribute to a workplace where individuals thrive, relationships deepen, and the journey toward success becomes both enriching and meaningful.

Recognizing and Validating Emotions in the Workplace:

The workplace is not just a space for tasks and projects; it's a melting pot of emotions. Here, we explore the art of recognizing and validating emotions in the workplace. It's about acknowledging that feelings, whether positive or challenging, are a natural part of the professional journey. By recognizing and validating the emotions of yourself and others, you contribute to a workplace culture that values authenticity and emotional well-being.

The workplace, contrary to a common misconception, is not a stoic arena devoid of emotions. It's a dynamic space where individuals experience a spectrum of feelings, from the highs of accomplishment to the challenges of setbacks. Recognizing and validating these emotions is akin to acknowledging the colors that paint the canvas of the professional journey.

Firstly, it involves self-awareness. Recognizing your own emotions, understanding their origins, and acknowledging their presence create a foundation for emotional intelligence. When individuals embrace their emotions without judgment, they pave the way for authenticity, allowing their true selves to shine through. This self-awareness becomes a guiding compass, influencing how one navigates challenges, communicates with others, and contributes to the collective emotional atmosphere.

Equally important is the ability to recognize and validate the emotions of others. This requires a keen sense of empathy—a skill that transcends mere sympathy and dives into a deep understanding of others' perspectives. It involves tuning in to the subtle cues of body language, facial expressions, and verbal signals. By recognizing when a colleague is excited about an achievement or struggling with a challenge, you create a culture that values each individual's emotional experience.

Validation, in this context, is the act of acknowledging and respecting the legitimacy of these emotions. It's about creating a space where individuals feel heard and understood, even when their emotions might differ from the prevailing tone. A workplace that validates emotions becomes a refuge—an environment where employees feel comfortable expressing their authentic selves without fear of judgment.

Why does this matter? The emotional well-being of individuals directly impacts their engagement, productivity, and overall job satisfaction. When emotions are recognized and validated, it fosters a culture of openness, trust, and camaraderie. It transforms the workplace from a mere professional setting to a community where individuals are seen not just as employees but as whole beings with varied emotional experiences.

Chapter Six

Adapting Communication Based on Others' Needs

Effective communication is a dance that adapts to the rhythm of others. This section delves into the heart of emotional intelligence—adapting communication based on the needs of those around you. It's about tuning in to the subtle cues of body language, tone, and unspoken messages. By understanding and adjusting your communication style, you create an environment where colleagues feel heard, understood, and valued.

Communication is more than words; it's a dance, a nuanced interplay of words, tone, and unspoken cues. In the dynamic landscape of the workplace, where individuals bring diverse experiences and perspectives, the ability to adapt communication based on the needs of others emerges as a cornerstone of emotional intelligence.

Consider communication as a musical composition, with each participant holding a unique instrument. Emotional intelligence is the conductor, orchestrating a harmonious symphony by attuning to the individual needs of each player. Here, we explore the transformative art of adapting communication, delving into the layers of understanding that contribute to a workplace culture where every voice is heard and valued.

At the heart of adapting communication is the recognition that individuals vary not only in their communication styles but also in how they receive and interpret messages. Some colleagues may appreciate direct and concise communication, while others may prefer a more conversational and contextual approach. Emotional intelligence prompts us to listen not just to the words spoken but to the subtle notes of body language, facial expressions, and the emotional undertones that accompany the message.

Adapting communication is about sensitivity to the unique needs of your audience. It involves recognizing when to provide detailed explanations and when to distill complex information into more accessible forms. It's a dance of empathy, where you attune your communication style to resonate with the emotions and preferences of those around you.

In practical terms, this might mean adjusting your tone and approach during a team meeting to ensure inclusivity. It could involve tailoring your written communication to suit the preferences of different team members. The art lies in being flexible, not rigid—in understanding that effective communication is a two-way street where the sender and receiver both play vital roles.

Adapting communication is not about manipulation or changing your authentic voice. It's about expanding your repertoire, much like a skilled dancer incorporating various styles into their routine. By embracing this fluidity, you create an environment where colleagues feel seen, heard, and understood. This, in turn, enhances collaboration, fosters a sense of belonging, and contributes to a workplace culture that thrives on effective and empathetic communication.

Embracing Vulnerability as Strength

In a world that often emphasizes strength as stoicism, this part explores the transformative power of embracing vulnerability. It's about recognizing that vulnerability is not a weakness but a profound strength. By being open about challenges, uncertainties, and even mistakes, you create a culture that fosters trust and authentic connections. Embracing vulnerability becomes a catalyst for personal and collective growth.

In the realm of the workplace, vulnerability is often viewed through the lens of fragility or weakness. However, a paradigm shift invites us to recognize vulnerability not as a liability but as an immense strength—a force that not only transforms individuals but also reshapes the very fabric of organizational culture.

The traditional view of vulnerability often associates it with exposure to harm or criticism. However, in the context of professional growth and relationships, vulnerability takes on a different hue. It is the courage to be authentic, transparent, and open about one's uncertainties, challenges, and even mistakes. It is an acknowledgment that, as professionals, we are not infallible, and embracing vulnerability becomes a conscious choice to connect with others on a human level.

When individuals in a workplace embrace vulnerability, it creates an environment that fosters trust and genuine connection. In a culture where colleagues feel safe to share their thoughts, concerns, and aspirations, relationships deepen, and collaboration flourishes. This authenticity becomes a catalyst for building a cohesive team where members support each other through challenges and celebrate victories together.

Vulnerability is intertwined with the willingness to learn and adapt. In an ever-evolving professional landscape, the ability to acknowledge gaps in knowledge or skills becomes a pathway to growth. When individuals feel secure enough to ask questions, seek guidance, or admit when they don't have all the answers, it paves the way for continuous learning and adaptation. Vulnerability, in this context, becomes the gateway to innovation and resilience.

Innovation often springs from spaces where individuals feel free to express unconventional ideas without fear of judgment. Embracing vulnerability nurtures a culture where creative thinking thrives. When professionals are encouraged to share their unique perspectives and take calculated risks without the fear of reprisal, it creates an environment ripe for innovation. Vulnerability becomes the driving force behind exploring new ideas and pushing the boundaries of what is possible.

In a workplace that embraces vulnerability, the stigma around mistakes diminishes. Instead, mistakes are viewed as opportunities for learning and improvement. The collective acknowledgment that everyone is on a journey of growth fosters a supportive culture where individuals lift each other up rather than tearing down. Vulnerability becomes the glue that binds a team together, creating a resilient and supportive professional community.

In conclusion, embracing vulnerability as strength is not a departure from professionalism; rather, it is an evolution. It is a recognition that true strength lies not in a facade of invulnerability but in the authentic expression of our human experiences. In a workplace that values vulnerability, individuals and teams flourish, innovation thrives, and success becomes a shared journey toward continuous improvement and excellence.

As we navigate the landscape of empathy and emotional intelligence, remember that these qualities are not just soft skills; they are the pillars that uphold a resilient and harmonious workplace culture. By recognizing emotions, adapting communication, and embracing vulnerability, you contribute to a professional environment where individuals thrive, relationships deepen, and success becomes a collective journey.

Chapter Seven

Mastering Interpersonal Relationships in the Workplace

In the intricate dance of the professional world, interpersonal relationships emerge as the choreography that defines success. This chapter is your guide to not only navigating but mastering the delicate art of human connections within the workplace. From collaborating with colleagues to building alliances that transcend cubicle boundaries, we delve into the nuances of interpersonal dynamics, unraveling the threads that weave a tapestry of trust, communication, and collaboration.

Before we embark on the journey of mastery, let's unravel the fabric of workplace relationships. They are not mere transactions; they are the heartbeat of a thriving professional ecosystem. Interpersonal relationships in the workplace extend beyond the confines of formal interactions—they encompass the unspoken cues, the shared laughter, and the genuine camaraderie that transforms colleagues into collaborators.

In this exploration, we dissect the anatomy of workplace relationships, recognizing that each interaction is an opportunity to forge a connection that transcends the transactional. From the mentorship that propels careers to the bonds formed in the crucible of shared challenges, we explore the diverse forms that workplace relationships can take and the transformative power they hold.

At the heart of every meaningful relationship lies trust—a currency that, once earned, becomes the cornerstone of collaboration. This section delves into the elements of trust, exploring how reliability, integrity, and transparency serve as the building blocks. We unravel the delicate dance of vulnerability and strength, understanding that trust is not just given; it's reciprocated through actions, consistency, and a shared commitment to mutual growth.

A workplace is a symphony of voices, ideas, and perspectives. Effective communication is the conductor that ensures harmony. In this segment, we explore the art of not just speaking but truly being heard. We navigate the nuances of verbal and non-verbal communication, understanding that it's not just about the words you say but how they resonate with others. From active listening to mastering the art of constructive feedback, we equip you with the tools to become a maestro in the symphony of workplace communication.

In the tapestry of workplace relationships, conflicts are the inevitable knots that demand attention. However, conflict is not the enemy; it's an opportunity for growth and understanding. This chapter provides a roadmap for navigating conflicts with finesse, transforming challenges into opportunities for stronger connections. We explore conflict resolution strategies, the art of compromise, and the importance of maintaining professionalism even in the face of disagreement.

A successful professional journey is not a solitary endeavor; it's a collaborative effort that thrives on networks. In this segment, we delve into the art of building a strategic network—from cultivating meaningful mentorships to forging alliances that amplify your impact. We discuss the dynamics of networking events, the power of genuine connections, and the importance of reciprocity in building a network that extends beyond LinkedIn connections.

Interpersonal mastery goes beyond the cognitive; it delves into the realm of emotional intelligence. This chapter explores the profound impact of understanding and managing emotions—both yours and others. From recognizing the emotional undercurrents in a negotiation to leading with empathy, we unravel the layers of emotional intelligence that elevate your ability to connect and collaborate.

As we traverse the chapters of "Mastering Interpersonal Relationships in the Workplace," remember that these skills are not just for professional survival but for thriving in the intricate ecosystem of your career. The workplace is not just a collection of desks and deadlines; it's a vibrant community of individuals, each with their strengths, aspirations, and stories. Mastery of interpersonal relationships is not just a skill; it's an investment in the richness and depth of your professional journey. So, let's dive into the intricacies, unravel the complexities, and emerge not just as professionals but as architects of meaningful connections in the tapestry of our careers.

Transitioning from Peer to Leader

The journey from being a peer to assuming a leadership role is a profound odyssey that reshapes not only one's professional identity but the entire dynamic of workplace relationships. As one steps into the shoes of a leader, the terrain changes, and the familiar landscape of camaraderie undergoes a transformation.

At the heart of this journey lie the challenges inherent in stepping up from a team member role. It's a shift that demands a recalibration of expectations, both from oneself and from those accustomed to seeing a colleague, not a leader. The familiarity of the team member's perspective evolves into the responsibility of making decisions that impact the entire group. It's not merely a promotion; it's a psychological shift that requires navigating potential resistance and embracing the discomfort of newfound authority.

Maintaining relationships while setting boundaries becomes the delicate artistry of this transition. The leader is no longer just a part of the team; they are now tasked with guiding and orchestrating the collective effort. This delicate balance involves preserving the trust and camaraderie established as peers while establishing the necessary boundaries that leadership demands. Clear communication becomes paramount, as does the ability to empathize with the team's evolving dynamics.

Embracing the responsibility of leadership is the keystone of this journey. It's more than wielding authority—it's about shouldering the weight of responsibility for the team's success and well-being. The leader becomes a facilitator, a guide, and a catalyst for growth. This shift in mindset involves viewing leadership not as a solo endeavor but as a collaborative effort where success is measured not just individually but by the collective achievements of the team.

The journey from peer to leader is a transformative process that goes beyond the confines of a new title. It's about mastering the intricate dance between authority and relatability, steering a team toward success while preserving the bonds forged in shared challenges. This journey is a testament to adaptability, resilience, and the ability to evolve not just professionally but personally. It's an exploration of leadership as a dynamic force, shaping not only the trajectory of a career but the very fabric of workplace relationships. As individuals embark on this transformative odyssey, they discover that being a leader is not just a destination—it's a continuous journey of growth, self-discovery, and the art of inspiring others to reach their full potential.

Challenges in stepping up from a team member role

Stepping into a leadership role brings a unique set of challenges, especially when transitioning from a familiar team member position. The dynamics shift, and suddenly, the once-equal relationships must adapt to the new hierarchy. This point delves into the intricacies of handling these challenges, acknowledging the potential resistance or discomfort that may accompany the elevation to a leadership position.

The transition from a team member to a leadership position is akin to navigating a shifting landscape, where familiarity gives way to new expectations and responsibilities. This metamorphosis is not without its challenges, and understanding and overcoming them is crucial for a seamless and effective transition.

One of the primary challenges is the subtle shift in dynamics within the team. As a team member, relationships are often characterized by a sense of equality and camaraderie. However, assuming a leadership role introduces a hierarchical element that can disrupt these established dynamics. Team members may grapple with adjusting to a new authority figure, and the leader, in turn, must navigate the fine line between being approachable and exercising necessary authority.

Another challenge lies in the potential resistance from team members who may view the transition with skepticism. The familiarity of the previous peer relationship can breed uncertainty or even resentment when one of their own assumes a leadership role. This resistance may manifest in subtle forms, such as reluctance to accept directives or a hesitancy to recognize the leader's newfound authority.

The shift in responsibilities is a significant hurdle. Team members turned leaders often find themselves juggling the demands of overseeing projects, making strategic decisions, and ensuring team cohesion. The skill set that made them an effective team member—be it technical expertise or a collaborative approach—must now expand to encompass leadership qualities such as strategic vision, decision-making prowess, and the ability to inspire and guide others.

Communication challenges also emerge during this transition. As a team member, communication is often horizontal, flowing seamlessly among peers. However, in a leadership role, effective communication requires a vertical dimension as directives and expectations are communicated downward. Leaders must adapt their communication style to convey authority while still fostering an open and collaborative environment.

Lastly, navigating the delicate balance between maintaining personal relationships and assuming a leadership role poses a challenge. Team members may struggle to reconcile the friendly peer they once knew with the authority figure now guiding the team. Leaders must find ways to preserve the positive aspects of their previous relationships while establishing the professional boundaries necessary for effective leadership.

In summary, the challenges in stepping up from a team member role are multifaceted. They encompass shifts in dynamics, potential resistance, expanded responsibilities, communication adjustments, and the delicate balance between friendship and leadership. Acknowledging and actively addressing these challenges is essential for a successful transition and the cultivation of a positive and productive leadership dynamic within the team.

Maintaining relationships while setting boundaries

Navigating the delicate balance between maintaining existing relationships and setting necessary boundaries is an art that effective leaders must master. This section explores strategies for fostering a collaborative environment while establishing the authority needed for effective leadership. It emphasizes the importance of clear communication and empathy to navigate this delicate tightrope.

One of the most delicate and nuanced aspects of transitioning from a peer to a leader is the art of maintaining relationships while simultaneously establishing necessary boundaries. It's akin to walking a tightrope, where balance and finesse become paramount.

In the realm of leadership, relationships are the backbone of a healthy and productive team. These relationships often have a history rooted in shared experiences, mutual support, and a sense of camaraderie. As one assumes a leadership role, the challenge lies in preserving these connections while redefining the parameters of interaction.

The key lies in transparent and empathetic communication. Leaders need to convey the shift in roles without undermining the value of existing relationships. It's about openly acknowledging the change, assuring team members that the foundation of trust and respect remains intact, and that the evolution is a natural progression.

Setting boundaries is not synonymous with creating barriers; it's about defining the expectations and structure essential for effective leadership. This involves clearly communicating roles, responsibilities, and decision-making processes. By articulating these boundaries, a leader ensures that the team understands the framework within which it operates.

Empathy plays a pivotal role in this delicate balancing act. Leaders need to appreciate that the transition might be challenging for team members who were once peers. They must be attuned to the potential feelings of uncertainty or even resistance. Addressing these concerns with empathy fosters an environment where team members feel heard and understood.

Additionally, leaders must lead by example. Demonstrating the ability to set boundaries without compromising interpersonal relationships sets the tone for the entire team. It shows that boundaries are not rigid barriers but guidelines that contribute to a more organized and efficient working environment.

Ultimately, maintaining relationships while setting boundaries is about preserving the heart of teamwork while adapting to the demands of leadership. It's about creating a workspace where professional relationships thrive within a framework of clarity and respect. This delicate dance requires a leader to be both assertive and understanding, firm yet flexible—a skill set that distinguishes exceptional leaders in the ever-evolving landscape of the workplace.

Embracing the responsibility of leadership

Assuming a leadership role goes beyond acquiring a new title—it's about embracing the weight of responsibility that comes with it. This point explores the mindset shift required to transition from an individual contributor to a leader. It emphasizes the transformative power of viewing leadership not as a position of authority but as an opportunity for personal and collective growth. Effective leadership is discussed not in terms of command and control but in terms of inspiration, guidance, and fostering an environment where the entire team can flourish.

Assuming a leadership role is more than a mere shift in title; it's a profound transformation that demands a recalibration of mindset and approach. In this section, we explore the essence of embracing the responsibility of leadership—a journey that transcends authority and embraces the true power of influence, guidance, and collective growth.

Leadership, at its core, is a commitment to something greater than oneself. It's a conscious decision to shoulder the responsibility not just for personal success but for the success and well-being of the entire team. Embracing the responsibility of leadership requires a departure from the notion that leadership is about dictating orders and exerting control. Instead, it's about becoming a facilitator, an enabler, and a source of inspiration for those you lead.

The mindset shift from an individual contributor to a leader involves recognizing that success is no longer measured solely by personal achievements but by the collective achievements of the team. It's an understanding that your role is not just to direct but to empower, not just to command but to inspire. This shift in perspective is akin to stepping onto a new landscape, one where the focus expands beyond immediate tasks to the long-term vision and growth of the team.

One crucial aspect of embracing leadership is cultivating a sense of ownership—not just of successes but also of failures. Leaders don't shy away from accountability; they embrace it. They understand that with authority comes responsibility, and with responsibility comes the inevitability of setbacks and challenges. Rather than viewing failures as roadblocks, effective leaders see them as opportunities for learning and improvement. This section delves into the importance of fostering a culture where taking ownership is not just encouraged but celebrated as a step toward progress.

Communication becomes a cornerstone in the journey of embracing leadership responsibility. It's not just about conveying directives; it's about fostering open and transparent communication channels. Leaders are effective communicators who listen as much as they speak, who value the input of their team, and who create an environment where ideas can flourish. This section provides insights into the art of communication that goes beyond conveying information to building connections and understanding within the team.

Furthermore, effective leadership involves the ability to adapt and evolve. Embracing responsibility means being agile in the face of change, acknowledging that the business landscape is dynamic, and being open to innovative approaches. Leaders become lifelong learners, constantly seeking opportunities for personal and professional development and encouraging their team to do the same.

Inclusive Leadership in a Diverse World

In an era where diversity is not just a buzzword but a cornerstone of success. It explores not only the importance of diverse perspectives but also the techniques leaders can employ to foster inclusivity in decision-making while avoiding the pitfalls of unconscious biases.

The importance of diverse perspectives cannot be overstated. In today's interconnected world, where the complexity of challenges demands multifaceted solutions, leaders must recognize the strategic advantage of incorporating a range of viewpoints. This part of the exploration dives into the transformative power of diversity, emphasizing that it's not just a matter of ticking boxes but a catalyst for innovation, adaptability, and holistic problem-solving. Inclusive leadership acknowledges that diversity is not a checkbox to be marked but an active pursuit of varied perspectives that enrich the collective intelligence of the team.

Moving beyond the theoretical, the discussion shifts to practical techniques for ensuring inclusivity in decision-making. Inclusivity is not a passive state but a deliberate practice, and this section provides leaders with actionable insights. From fostering an environment where every voice is heard to implementing structures that guarantee equitable participation, leaders are equipped with the tools to make inclusivity a tangible and integral part of their leadership approach.

However, the path to inclusive leadership is fraught with the subtleties of unconscious biases. Unraveling these biases is not just about recognizing them; it's about actively mitigating their impact. Leaders are guided through strategies to create awareness, foster continuous learning, and instill a sense of accountability within the team. By doing so, they cultivate a culture where decisions are rooted in merit rather than preconceived notions, ensuring that inclusivity is not compromised by hidden biases.

In a nutshell, this exploration of inclusive leadership is a call to action. It challenges leaders to move beyond rhetoric and actively champion diversity not just as a corporate value but as a guiding principle in their decision-making, team dynamics, and overall leadership philosophy. In a diverse world, inclusive leadership is not just a virtue; it's a strategic imperative that empowers teams to thrive amid the richness of differences.

Importance of diverse perspectives

The journey toward inclusive leadership begins with a profound understanding of the significance of diverse perspectives. This section delves into the transformative power of embracing a variety of viewpoints, experiences, and backgrounds within a team. Leaders are guided through the exploration of how diversity is not just an ethical imperative but a strategic advantage, fostering innovation, resilience, and a deeper understanding of the multifaceted challenges and opportunities in the modern professional landscape.

In the modern workplace, the call for diversity is not just an ethical imperative but a strategic necessity. The importance of diverse perspectives is akin to infusing a breath of fresh air into the corporate ecosystem, propelling organizations toward innovation, adaptability, and sustainable growth.

Diverse perspectives bring with them a richness that goes beyond the surface-level demographics of a team. It's about harnessing the unique experiences, cultural backgrounds, and ways of thinking that each individual brings to the table. In a world marked by rapid change and complexity, a team comprised of diverse perspectives becomes a powerhouse of creativity and resilience.

Innovation thrives in an environment where multiple lenses are applied to a challenge. A team with varied perspectives is better equipped to approach problems from different angles, uncovering solutions that might elude a more homogenous group. This diversity of thought becomes a catalyst for groundbreaking ideas, pushing organizations to the forefront of their industries.

Moreover, diverse perspectives enhance adaptability. In an era where change is constant, the ability to pivot and evolve is a critical factor for success. A team that represents a spectrum of backgrounds is inherently more adaptable, as its members bring a variety of insights and approaches to navigate the complexities of a dynamic marketplace.

Beyond the tangible benefits, fostering diverse perspectives in the workplace is a reflection of an organization's commitment to fairness, equality, and inclusion. It sends a powerful message that every voice matters, regardless of gender, ethnicity, or background. This inclusivity not only boosts morale but also attracts top talent, as individuals seek workplaces that value and celebrate their uniqueness.

Thus, the importance of diverse perspectives is a recognition that the challenges of today's professional landscape demand a tapestry of ideas, experiences, and approaches. It's about creating a workplace where diversity is not just a checkbox on a corporate agenda but an integral part of the organizational DNA. As organizations embrace and champion diverse perspectives, they not only fortify their present but lay the foundation for a future marked by innovation, resilience, and sustained success.

Techniques to ensure inclusivity in decision-making

Inclusivity is not a passive state but an active practice, especially in decision-making. Here, leaders are equipped with practical techniques to ensure that decision-making processes are inclusive. This involves creating an environment where all voices are heard, valuing input from diverse team members, and implementing structures that ensure equitable participation. From embracing collaborative decision-making models to leveraging technology for inclusive feedback, this section provides actionable insights for leaders committed to making inclusivity a guiding principle in their leadership journey.

In the intricate dance of leadership, decision-making stands as a pivotal act that shapes the trajectory of a team. Ensuring inclusivity in this process is not merely a noble aspiration; it's a strategic imperative that elevates the collective intelligence of the team and fosters an environment where diverse perspectives are not just heard but actively valued.

One of the foundational techniques in promoting inclusivity in decision-making is embracing a collaborative approach. Leaders are encouraged to shift from a top-down decision-making model to one that involves team members at various levels. This not only widens the pool of perspectives but also creates a sense of ownership among the team. Collaborative decision-making is not about relinquishing authority but about leveraging the collective wisdom of the team to make well-informed choices.

Another crucial technique involves creating structured spaces for inclusive discussions. This goes beyond casual brainstorming sessions to intentionally designed forums where team members feel empowered to voice their opinions. Leaders can implement techniques such as round-robin discussions, where every team member has an opportunity to contribute without fear of interruption, and anonymous feedback channels, allowing individuals to share perspectives without the burden of personal attribution.

Leveraging technology is a contemporary technique that leaders can employ to ensure inclusivity in decision-making. Virtual collaboration tools, survey platforms, and feedback mechanisms provide avenues for team members to contribute irrespective of their physical location or hierarchical position. This not only democratizes the decision-making process but also accommodates the preferences and working styles of diverse team members.

Moreover, leaders must be vigilant in recognizing and mitigating power dynamics that can hinder inclusivity. Techniques such as rotating leadership roles in decision-making meetings, actively seeking input from quieter team members, and employing structured decision-making frameworks contribute to a more level playing field.

Chapter Eight

Avoiding unconscious biases

Even the most well-intentioned leaders can be influenced by unconscious biases that impact decision-making. This part of the book delves into the nuanced world of unconscious biases—those subtle, automatic judgments that can unintentionally influence our perceptions. Leaders are guided through strategies to recognize and mitigate these biases, fostering an environment where decisions are made based on merit rather than preconceived notions. The emphasis is on creating a culture of awareness, continuous learning, and accountability to ensure that inclusivity is not undermined by hidden biases.

At the heart of avoiding unconscious biases lies the acknowledgment that they exist. Leaders must embark on a journey of self-awareness, fostering an environment where they recognize and confront their own biases. This involves embracing discomfort, challenging assumptions, and actively seeking diverse perspectives to counteract the automatic judgments that may arise.

Furthermore, leaders are guided to implement strategies that interrupt the influence of unconscious biases in decision-making processes. This includes adopting objective criteria for evaluation, implementing blind recruitment practices, and establishing structures that promote transparency and accountability. By consciously designing processes that minimize the impact of biases, leaders create a level playing field where merit takes precedence over preconceived notions.

Education becomes a powerful tool in the arsenal against unconscious biases. Leaders are encouraged to invest in ongoing learning initiatives that not only enhance their understanding of diversity and inclusion but also equip their teams with the tools to recognize and address biases collectively. By fostering a culture of continuous education, leaders ensure that unconscious biases are not just acknowledged but actively dismantled.

Ultimately, avoiding unconscious biases is not a one-time task but a commitment to ongoing vigilance. Leaders must be attuned to the evolving dynamics of their teams and the broader professional landscape. They are urged to create open channels of communication where team members feel empowered to raise awareness about potential biases and contribute to a culture of collective accountability.

In the pursuit of avoiding unconscious biases, leaders transform not only their decision-making processes but also the very fabric of their organizational culture. It's a conscious choice to build a workplace where diversity is not just welcomed but celebrated, and where every individual, regardless of background or identity, can thrive based on their merits and contributions.

Strategies for Effective Decision-Making

Effective decision-making is the cornerstone of successful leadership. Effective decision-making is the compass that guides leaders through the intricate landscape of leadership. It's not just about making choices; it's about making choices that align with the overarching vision, values, and goals of the organization. In this exploration of strategies for effective decision-making, we unravel the threads that elevate decisions from routine tasks to impactful contributions.

One critical facet of effective decision-making is embracing analytical approaches. Leaders are encouraged to view decision-making as a methodical process, leveraging data-driven tools such as SWOT analyses and cost-benefit assessments. By adopting this structured approach, leaders transform decisions into strategic moves, grounded in evidence and foresight.

However, effective decision-making goes beyond numbers and metrics; it involves striking a delicate balance between data and intuition. Leaders are urged to trust their instincts, drawing on their wealth of experience to complement quantitative analyses. This fusion of the analytical and the intuitive creates a decision-making process that is both informed and responsive to the dynamic nature of the professional landscape.

The journey of effective decision-making doesn't end with the choice itself; it extends to the proactive management of decision repercussions. Every decision, no matter how well-considered, has consequences. Leaders are guided through the art of anticipating potential outcomes, developing contingency plans, and fostering adaptability within their teams. By taking ownership of both decisions and their repercussions, leaders transform challenges into opportunities for growth and improvement.

Analytical Approaches to Decision-Making

This section unravels the power of analytical thinking in the decision-making process. Leaders are guided through the methodologies of data-driven decision-making, emphasizing the importance of gathering and analyzing relevant information.

At the heart of analytical decision-making lies a commitment to gathering, interpreting, and leveraging relevant information. Leaders are encouraged to adopt systematic methodologies such as SWOT analyses, cost-benefit assessments, and risk evaluations to illuminate the landscape before them. This structured approach ensures that decisions are not driven by impulse but by a comprehensive understanding of the variables at play.

Data-driven decision-making isn't merely about drowning in a sea of numbers; it's about extracting actionable insights. Leaders are guided through the process of identifying key performance indicators (KPIs) and leveraging data to gain insights into market trends, customer behavior, and internal operations. This strategic deployment of data transforms information from a mere resource to a powerful tool for making decisions that are not just timely but strategic.

Moreover, analytical approaches provide a framework for evaluating options objectively. By establishing clear criteria for decision-making, leaders can compare alternatives based on quantifiable metrics, minimizing the impact of personal biases. This objectivity ensures that decisions align with organizational goals and contribute to the overarching strategy.

The beauty of analytical decision-making lies in its adaptability. Leaders are equipped to navigate uncertainty by continuously monitoring and reassessing data. In a rapidly evolving business landscape, this adaptability becomes a superpower, enabling leaders to respond proactively to emerging challenges and opportunities.

Balancing Data with Intuition

While analytics provide a robust foundation, effective decision-making involves more than just numbers. Leaders are encouraged to embrace the art of balancing data with intuition. This involves tapping into their wealth of experience, leveraging gut instincts, and recognizing the human factor in decision-making. By striking a harmonious balance between quantitative analysis and intuitive understanding, leaders elevate their decision-making prowess to a level that transcends mere calculations.

Data, the bedrock of analytical decision-making, offers a tangible and quantifiable foundation. Leaders are encouraged to harness the power of data analytics, leveraging tools and methodologies to extract meaningful insights. Whether it's interpreting market trends, evaluating performance metrics, or conducting a comprehensive risk analysis, data-driven decision-making provides a structured approach to navigate the complexities of the business landscape.

Yet, effective decision-making is not confined to the realm of spreadsheets and algorithms. The human dimension, with its nuances and unpredictabilities, introduces a vital element that cannot be entirely captured by data alone. This is where intuition steps into the spotlight. Intuition, honed through experience and a deep understanding of the industry and team dynamics, allows leaders to tap into a reservoir of tacit knowledge. It's the gut feeling, the sixth sense, that complements the stark numbers and charts with a more holistic understanding of the situation.

The art lies in finding the synergy between data and intuition. Leaders are urged to avoid the extremes—neither dismissing the cold, hard facts nor relying solely on gut feelings. Instead, it's about recognizing the strengths of each approach and seamlessly integrating them into the decision-making process. This involves acknowledging when the data is insufficient and intuition is paramount, as well as when data should take precedence over gut feelings.

Balancing data with intuition is not a static formula but a dynamic dance that requires continuous refinement. It's an ongoing process of learning, adapting, and understanding the evolving landscape of the industry and the organization. By mastering this delicate equilibrium, leaders transcend the confines of rigid decision-making frameworks, navigating the complexity of the business world with a finesse that combines the precision of science with the artistry of intuition.

Managing the Repercussions of Decisions

Every decision, no matter how well-informed, carries repercussions. This section navigates the strategies leaders can employ to manage and mitigate the impact of their decisions. It involves anticipating potential outcomes, developing contingency plans, and fostering a culture of adaptability. Leaders are guided through the importance of not only making sound decisions but also taking ownership of their repercussions, transforming challenges into opportunities for growth and improvement.

Central to this exploration is the recognition that decisions, even well-considered ones, carry consequences. Leaders are guided through strategies to anticipate potential outcomes, fostering a foresight that empowers them to navigate the complex landscape of repercussions. This involves developing contingency plans, considering alternative scenarios, and embracing a proactive stance to address challenges that may arise.

Moreover, effective leaders understand the importance of taking ownership of the repercussions of their decisions. They recognize that leadership is not just about making choices but also about being accountable for the outcomes. This section encourages leaders to foster a culture of transparency and openness, where team members feel informed and engaged in understanding the implications of decisions.

Ultimately, managing the repercussions of decisions is not about avoiding challenges but about transforming them into opportunities for growth and improvement. It involves the resilience to adapt to unforeseen circumstances, the agility to course-correct when needed, and the wisdom to view setbacks not as failures but as stepping stones toward organizational evolution.

Leading During Crisis

In the crucible of leadership, the ability to steer a team through turbulent times is a hallmark of true leadership. In the fast-paced and unpredictable landscape of the corporate world, leaders often find themselves navigating uncharted territories during crises. Leading effectively in times of turmoil is an art that transcends traditional leadership skills, demanding a unique blend of resilience, composure, and a profound commitment to the well-being of the team.

The cornerstone of leading during a crisis is the ability to stay calm under pressure. In the corporate realm, where decisions have a domino effect on the entire organization, leaders must exude a sense of stability even in the face of uncertainty. This involves managing stress, making strategic decisions with a clear mind, and projecting an unwavering confidence that becomes a source of reassurance for the team.

Communication emerges as a linchpin ineffective leadership during a crisis. The corporate world is interconnected, and during turbulent times, information becomes a lifeline. Leaders must master the art of communicating with clarity and transparency, keeping the team informed about developments, addressing concerns promptly, and providing a roadmap even when the path is foggy. Effective communication fosters trust and unity, critical elements for navigating the complexities of a corporate crisis.

Rallying the team and maintaining morale is another facet of leading during a crisis in the corporate world. The impact of a crisis extends beyond the bottom line; it permeates the morale and spirit of the team. Leaders must inspire and motivate, instilling a collective sense of purpose that transcends the challenges at hand. This involves acknowledging individual contributions, fostering a culture of support, and demonstrating a steadfast commitment to overcoming adversity together.

Staying Calm Under Pressure

Leadership is often tested in the crucible of crisis, where the stakes are high, and pressure is relentless. This section explores the importance of maintaining a calm demeanor as a leader, regardless of the storm swirling around. Leaders are guided through strategies for managing stress, making informed decisions under pressure, and projecting an aura of stability that becomes a guiding light for the team.

Staying calm under pressure is not merely a stoic facade; it's a strategic imperative. Leaders who can maintain composure amidst chaos exhibit a form of resilience that becomes a guiding force for the entire team. In the corporate world, where decisions are magnified and ripple effects are felt across departments, the leader's ability to manage stress becomes a critical factor in steering the ship through turbulent waters.

This skill involves a multifaceted approach. It begins with self-awareness—an understanding of one's triggers and stressors. Leaders are encouraged to cultivate mindfulness practices that allow them to stay present and focused even when the stakes are high. Additionally, effective leaders recognize the importance of seeking support, whether through mentorship, peer collaboration, or external resources. The ability to share the burden of decision-making and seek guidance when needed contributes to sustained composure.

Strategic decision-making is at the core of staying calm under pressure. Leaders are guided through methodologies that help them make informed choices even in high-pressure situations. This involves prioritizing tasks, breaking down complex problems into manageable components, and maintaining a strategic vision that transcends immediate challenges.

Ultimately, staying calm under pressure is not just about managing the external circumstances; it's about mastering the internal landscape. Leaders who cultivate a calm and focused mindset become beacons of stability for their teams. In the whirlwind of corporate challenges, this trait is not just a leadership skill; it's a transformative force that elevates decision-making, fosters a resilient team culture, and positions the organization for sustained success.

Effective Communication During Turbulence

Communication is the lifeblood of effective leadership, and during a crisis, it becomes even more pivotal.

Clarity is paramount in effective communication during workplace turbulence. Leaders must provide clear and concise information about the situation, ensuring that the team comprehends the intricacies of the challenges at hand. Ambiguity breeds anxiety, and in times of uncertainty, clarity becomes a beacon that guides the team through the storm. Transparent communication builds trust, assuring team members that they are informed and valued contributors to the collective journey.

Empathy is the soul of effective communication during turbulence. Leaders must recognize the emotional toll that uncertainty can take on individuals within the organization. This involves not only addressing concerns and fears but also demonstrating a genuine understanding of the human aspect of the challenges. Empathetic communication creates a culture of solidarity, where team members feel seen, heard, and supported, fostering a collective sense of resilience.

Timeliness is a strategic element in the communication arsenal during turbulence. In a rapidly changing landscape, delays in information can lead to confusion and mistrust. Leaders must adopt an agile approach, providing updates and guidance in a timely manner. This involves leveraging communication channels efficiently, whether through team meetings, email updates, or other platforms that ensure information flows seamlessly.

Moreover, effective communication during workplace turbulence extends beyond the spoken or written word. Non-verbal cues, such as body language and tone, play a significant role in conveying messages. Leaders must be mindful of these nuances, ensuring that their demeanor aligns with the messages they convey, reinforcing a sense of stability and confidence within the team.

Rallying the Team and Maintaining Morale

A crisis can shake the very foundation of a team's morale, and effective leaders understand the delicate task of rallying the troops. This section provides insights into the strategies leaders can employ to inspire and motivate the team during challenging times. It involves fostering a sense of unity, acknowledging individual contributions, and instilling a collective sense of purpose that becomes a beacon of hope in the midst of adversity.

The workplace is not just a collection of individuals performing tasks; it's a community, a collective force that thrives on collaboration and shared purpose. When faced with challenges, effective leaders understand the nuanced art of rallying the team and maintaining morale, recognizing that the spirit of the workforce is a driving force behind resilience and success.

Maintaining morale is more than a superficial boost in team spirit; it's an investment in the emotional well-being and engagement of each team member. Leaders play a pivotal role in creating an environment where individuals feel not only valued for their contributions but also supported during challenging times. This involves acknowledging the efforts of each team member, fostering a culture of appreciation, and providing avenues for personal and professional growth.

During times of adversity, effective leaders become architects of inspiration. They understand that maintaining morale is not about downplaying challenges but about instilling a collective sense of purpose that transcends difficulties. This involves transparent communication, where leaders share the broader vision, the steps being taken to address challenges, and the crucial role each team member plays in the journey.

Rallying the team goes beyond motivational speeches; it's about creating a culture of collaboration and support. Leaders foster an environment where team members feel connected to a shared mission, where the success of one is celebrated as the success of all. This involves recognizing individual strengths, encouraging collaboration, and fostering a sense of camaraderie that transforms the workplace into a community of resilience.

Continuous Learning and Adaptability

In the dynamic landscape of the professional world, the journey of leadership is intertwined with the ethos of continuous learning and adaptability.

The importance of continuous learning is rooted in the dynamic nature of industries. In a world where technological advancements, market shifts, and global changes are constant, those who cease to learn risk becoming obsolete. Leaders who embrace a mindset of continuous learning position themselves as agile navigators, capable of steering through uncertainties with the latest insights and skills. Moreover, this commitment sets a powerful example for their teams, fostering a culture of curiosity and growth.

Adaptability is the twin pillar that complements continuous learning. The ability to pivot, innovate, and thrive amidst change is a hallmark of successful individuals and organizations. In the workplace, adaptability is not just about reacting to external changes; it's about proactively anticipating and shaping them. Leaders who embody adaptability inspire resilience within their teams, creating an environment where challenges are viewed not as obstacles but as opportunities for creative solutions and growth.

Continuous learning and adaptability are not isolated endeavors; they are interconnected facets of a growth-oriented mindset. Seeking feedback and engaging in self-assessment are integral components of this journey. Leaders who actively seek feedback demonstrate a commitment to improvement, turning each piece of critique into a stepping stone toward excellence. Self-assessment becomes a reflective practice, allowing leaders to identify areas of growth and refine their approaches.

Furthermore, encouraging a culture of learning within the team is not just about providing training programs; it's about fostering an environment where curiosity is celebrated, mistakes are viewed as learning experiences, and innovation is a shared goal. In such a culture, teams become dynamic, resilient entities capable of navigating change with enthusiasm and creativity.

Importance of Ongoing Professional Development

Leadership is not a static position but a continuous journey of growth. This section explores the significance of ongoing professional development for leaders. It emphasizes the commitment to staying abreast of industry trends, acquiring new skills, and evolving as a leader in tandem with the changing professional landscape. The pursuit of knowledge becomes not just a task but a mindset—an understanding that stagnation is the antithesis of effective leadership.

The pace of change in industries today is unparalleled, driven by technological advancements, market dynamics, and the evolving needs of consumers. In this ever-shifting landscape, leaders are not just stewards of their current roles; they are navigators of change, requiring a skill set that adapts to emerging challenges. Ongoing professional development is the key to unlocking this adaptive potential.

The rapid evolution of skills and knowledge necessitates a commitment to staying abreast of industry trends. Ongoing professional development is a proactive response to this necessity, ensuring that leaders remain not only relevant but also ahead of the curve. It transforms the workplace into a dynamic ecosystem where learning becomes a continuous, integrated part of the professional journey.

Moreover, the commitment to ongoing professional development is a powerful catalyst for individual and collective growth. It cultivates a culture of curiosity, resilience, and a thirst for excellence. Leaders who prioritize continuous learning set a precedent for their teams, creating an environment where skill enhancement is not just encouraged but expected.

In the realm of leadership, ongoing professional development is not merely about acquiring new skills; it's about honing the ability to think critically, adapt swiftly, and lead with foresight. It's an investment in the intellectual capital of the workforce, a recognition that the strength of an organization lies not just in its present capabilities but in its capacity to evolve.

Seeking Feedback and Self-Assessment

Leadership is a journey of self-discovery and refinement. Here, leaders are guided through the art of seeking feedback and engaging in self-assessment. This involves fostering an open feedback culture where constructive criticism is viewed not as a criticism but as a catalyst for improvement. Leaders are encouraged to engage in reflective practices, recognizing that self-awareness is the foundation of personal and professional growth.

Leadership is, at its essence, a dynamic journey of growth and refinement. Seeking feedback from peers, team members, and mentors serves as a compass in this journey. Constructive feedback is not a critique of one's abilities but a mirror reflecting areas of strength and areas for improvement. Leaders who actively seek feedback are not only open to refinement but demonstrate a commitment to understanding the impact of their actions on those they lead.

Self-assessment goes hand in hand with seeking external feedback. It involves a deep dive into one's own leadership style, decision-making processes, and interpersonal dynamics. This introspective practice is not about self-criticism but about fostering self-awareness—the bedrock of effective leadership. Leaders engaged in self-assessment recognize their strengths, acknowledge their limitations, and proactively seek opportunities for growth.

The importance of seeking feedback and self-assessment extends beyond individual development to the broader organizational context. Leaders who embrace these practices contribute to a culture of openness and continuous improvement. Team members, witnessing their leaders actively engaging in self-reflection, are encouraged to do the same. It becomes a collective journey toward excellence, where feedback is not perceived as a threat but as a valuable resource for the entire team's advancement.

Encouraging a Culture of Learning within the Team

The ethos of continuous learning extends beyond individual leaders to the collective team. This section provides insights into strategies for leaders to encourage a culture of learning within their teams. It involves creating opportunities for skill development, providing resources for ongoing education, and fostering an environment where curiosity and innovation are celebrated. In a culture of learning, challenges become opportunities, and each team member is empowered to contribute their unique strengths to the collective growth.

Encouraging a culture of learning within the team is an investment in the team's adaptability and resilience. In the fast-paced professional landscape, where change is constant, a learning culture positions the team not as mere responders to challenges but as proactive agents of innovation. It creates a mindset where challenges are viewed as opportunities for growth and where the team collectively engages in a continuous journey of improvement.

Moreover, a culture of learning enhances the overall skill set and versatility of the team. By providing resources, training opportunities, and platforms for skill development, leaders empower team members to expand their capabilities. This not only enhances individual contributions but also creates a dynamic and versatile team that can navigate diverse challenges with agility.

In a culture of learning, curiosity is celebrated, and experimentation is encouraged. It fosters an environment where team members feel not only free but inspired to explore new ideas, technologies, and methodologies. This freedom of exploration becomes a wellspring of innovation, where novel solutions to complex problems emerge from a team that embraces the joy of learning.

Furthermore, a learning culture contributes to employee engagement and satisfaction. When team members feel that their growth and development are valued, they are more likely to be motivated, committed, and satisfied in their roles. It creates a positive feedback loop where engaged employees contribute to a thriving culture of learning, further fueling the team's collective success.

Chapter Nine

Branding Yourself: Your Professional Identity

In the vast and competitive landscape of the professional world, your personal brand is the compass that not only guides your journey but also leaves an indelible mark on those who encounter it. In this chapter, we embark on a journey of self-discovery and strategic self-presentation, exploring the art and science of branding yourself in a way that resonates with authenticity and captivates the attention of your professional audience.

Your professional identity is more than a resume or a LinkedIn profile—it's a narrative that defines who you are, what you stand for, and the value you bring to the table. Personal branding is not a vanity exercise; it's a strategic investment in your career. As the saying goes,

"Your brand is what people say about you when you're not in the room." In a world inundated with information and choices, your personal brand serves as a beacon, guiding others in forming impressions and decisions about you.

In this section, we delve into the nuances of crafting a narrative that is not only compelling but also authentic. We explore the intersection of passion, expertise, and uniqueness—the sweet spot where your individuality shines. Through a series of exercises and reflections, you'll uncover the elements that define your professional story and distinguish you from the crowd. Whether you're a seasoned executive or an entry-level professional, the principles of narrative crafting are universal, and adapt to every stage of your career.

In the digital age, your online presence is often the first impression you make. From optimizing your LinkedIn profile to curating a professional online persona, we explore the strategies that amplify your brand in the virtual realm. We discuss the do's and don'ts of social media, the art of storytelling in a digital format, and how to leverage online platforms to showcase your expertise and connect with industry influencers.

A personal brand is not just about what you say; it's about what you do. In this section, we delve into the importance of authenticity in actions. We discuss the alignment of your professional values with your day-to-day behavior, exploring how consistency in your actions reinforces the authenticity of your brand. From networking events to daily interactions in the workplace, we uncover the subtle yet powerful ways in which your behavior shapes perceptions.

Your personal brand is dynamic, evolving with your growth and experiences. However, rebranding can be a delicate process, and setbacks can test the resilience of even the most meticulously crafted brand. In this section, we address the challenges of rebranding and provide strategies for overcoming setbacks. Whether you're transitioning to a new role, recovering from a professional misstep, or simply evolving in your career, this chapter equips you with the tools to navigate change with grace and purpose.

How do you know if your personal brand is making the desired impact? We introduce the concept of key performance indicators (KPIs) for personal branding—quantifiable metrics that help you assess the effectiveness of your brand strategy. From increased engagement on professional platforms to tangible career advancements, we explore the measurable outcomes that indicate your brand's influence and resonance.

Your personal brand extends beyond the confines of your current position or project. It's a legacy in the making, a narrative that transcends individual achievements. In this concluding section, we explore the concept of cultivating a lasting legacy through your professional identity. We discuss the principles of mentorship, knowledge sharing, and community engagement as avenues to leave a positive and enduring impact on the professional landscape.

Understanding Personal Branding

Personal branding is the art and science of curating a distinct and memorable image that encapsulates who you are, what you stand for, and the unique value you bring to the professional arena. It's not just a logo or a tagline; it's a holistic representation of your professional identity, a narrative that extends beyond your resume and permeates every interaction and engagement in your career.

At its core, personal branding matters because in a world saturated with information, impressions are formed swiftly, and attention spans are limited. Your personal brand is the shorthand version of your professional story—the quick snapshot that influences how others perceive and engage with you. In the vast and interconnected landscape of the professional world, a strong personal brand is your strategic advantage.

Personal branding is a powerful tool for individuals navigating the corporate world, acting as a strategic compass in the dynamic sea of professional interactions. In an era where first impressions often occur online, a well-crafted personal brand serves as a virtual handshake, making an immediate and lasting impact. It's not merely a self-promotion tactic but a means of communicating one's unique value proposition and professional identity.

In the competitive landscape of the corporate world, personal branding distinguishes individuals from their peers. It shapes perceptions, establishes credibility, and opens doors to opportunities. A strong personal brand is a career asset, influencing career progression, job prospects, and even the ability to negotiate favorable terms. It's a testament to one's expertise, reliability, and leadership potential.

Moreover, personal branding is a proactive approach to professional development. By intentionally shaping how one is perceived, individuals can align their brand with their career aspirations. It fosters authenticity, allowing professionals to showcase not only their skills but also their values and passions. In a corporate environment that values both competence and character, personal branding becomes a strategic investment that pays dividends in career growth and fulfillment. Ultimately, personal branding empowers individuals to take control of their narrative, stand out in a crowded marketplace, and navigate the complexities of the corporate world with confidence and purpose.

Differentiating between personal and professional identities is a crucial aspect of understanding personal branding. While your professional identity encompasses your skills, experiences, and qualifications, your personal brand adds a layer of humanity to this equation.

It's the unique blend of your personality, values, and passions that distinguishes you from a sea of similarly qualified professionals. Personal branding bridges the gap between the technical proficiency listed on your resume and the person behind the professional facade.

Differentiating between personal and professional identities is paramount in the realm of personal branding as it delineates the multifaceted dimensions of an individual. While the professional identity encapsulates qualifications, skills, and work-related accomplishments, the personal brand adds a human touch, revealing the unique amalgamation of one's personality, values, and passions. This distinction is vital because it transforms a mere list of professional achievements into a relatable and authentic narrative.

In a competitive professional landscape, where technical skills are often comparable, personal branding becomes the differentiator. It allows individuals to stand out by showcasing not only what they do but who they are. The personal brand becomes a magnetic force, attracting opportunities, collaborations, and meaningful connections.

Moreover, by acknowledging and nurturing the personal aspects of identity, professionals can establish a more profound and lasting impact. Clients, colleagues, and employers are not just engaging with a set of skills; they are connecting with a person—an individual with a story, a vision, and a set of values. This deeper connection fosters trust, loyalty, and a sense of authenticity, which are invaluable assets in the professional world.

Consistency across all touchpoints is the glue that holds your personal brand together. Whether it's your LinkedIn profile, a networking event, or a presentation at work, each touchpoint is an opportunity to reinforce your brand identity. Consistency doesn't mean uniformity; it means maintaining a cohesive narrative and visual identity that aligns with your overarching brand strategy. From the language you use in emails to the way you present yourself in meetings, each touchpoint contributes to the cumulative image of your personal brand.

Digital Footprint and Online Presence

In the age of connectivity, your digital footprint is the echo of your professional existence. LinkedIn, in particular, acts as a nexus for corporate professionals, offering a platform to showcase not just qualifications but thought leadership, industry engagement, and a collaborative spirit. The interconnected nature of professional networks creates a web of opportunities, enabling individuals to stay abreast of industry trends, connect with like-minded professionals, and position themselves as leaders in their field.

Balancing personal and professional content online is crucial. While expertise and achievements are paramount, injecting elements of your personality and interests humanizes your professional image. This balance fosters genuine connections, enhancing your relatability and influencing potential collaborations.

Moreover, a strategic online reputation is a valuable asset in the corporate realm. Employers and colleagues often conduct online due diligence, and a positive online reputation enhances trust, credibility, and professional influence. As the corporate world becomes increasingly digital, individuals who understand and master the nuances of their digital footprint and online presence gain a competitive edge, creating a narrative that resonates and propels them toward continuous success.

Importance of LinkedIn and Other Professional Networks

LinkedIn, often regarded as the digital headquarters of professionals, plays a pivotal role in shaping your online presence. It serves as a dynamic virtual resume, showcasing not just your professional journey but also providing a platform for networking, thought leadership, and industry engagement. Beyond LinkedIn, other professional networks contribute to the expansion of your digital footprint, creating a web of connections and opportunities that transcend geographical boundaries. The interconnected nature of these platforms amplifies your reach and influence within the professional community.

LinkedIn and other professional networks serve as the cornerstone of an impactful digital footprint, holding the potential to shape and elevate your online presence in the professional sphere. LinkedIn, often hailed as the virtual resume of the modern professional, acts as a dynamic showcase of your skills, experiences, and professional journey. It goes beyond the static details of a traditional resume, fostering engagement, networking, and thought leadership within a global community of professionals.

The importance of these platforms lies not only in the presentation of your credentials but also in the opportunities they create. Networking transcends geographical boundaries, providing avenues for collaboration, mentorship, and career advancement. Through these networks, professionals can actively participate in industry conversations, stay abreast of trends, and position themselves as thought leaders, amplifying their influence within their respective fields.

Moreover, professional networks contribute to the interconnected web of digital footprints. They serve as nodes in a vast ecosystem, where each connection and interaction adds layers to your online persona. In the digital age, where visibility is a currency, these platforms provide a stage to showcase expertise, build meaningful relationships, and leave a lasting impact on the professional landscape.

Balancing Personal and Professional Content Online

Maintaining a delicate equilibrium between personal and professional content is an art form in the digital realm. While showcasing your expertise is crucial, offering glimpses into your personality and interests adds a human touch to your online persona. Striking this balance is about being authentic and relatable, sharing insights from your professional journey while also showcasing the diverse facets of your life. This authenticity fosters a connection that goes beyond the transactional, building relationships based on shared values and interests.

In the corporate world's digital landscape, balancing personal and professional content online is akin to orchestrating a symphony that harmonizes competence with relatability. While showcasing professional achievements is integral for credibility, injecting personal elements into your online presence adds depth and authenticity. It humanizes the digital persona, fostering connections beyond the transactional and creating an environment where relationships are built on shared values and interests.

The importance of this equilibrium lies in the power to forge meaningful connections. Colleagues, clients, and industry peers are not just interacting with a list of accomplishments; they are engaging with a person. Personal content serves as the glue that binds professional relationships, transcending the boundaries of formalities and fostering a sense of camaraderie.

Moreover, in a corporate world that increasingly values diversity and inclusion, showcasing personal aspects online contributes to a more holistic representation. It breaks down the traditional walls that separate professional and personal spheres, fostering a workplace culture where individuals are recognized not just for their skills but for the richness of their experiences and perspectives.

Strategies to Enhance Online Reputation

Your online reputation is a currency in the digital economy. This section delves into actionable strategies to not only enhance but also protect your online reputation. From crafting a compelling LinkedIn profile to actively engaging in industry conversations, each online interaction contributes to your reputation. Moreover, we explore the importance of proactive reputation management, addressing and mitigating any potential pitfalls that may arise. The digital landscape is both a showcase and a stage, and understanding how to navigate it strategically is paramount for building a positive and influential online reputation.

Crafting a compelling LinkedIn profile serves as the digital gateway to your professional persona, offering a snapshot of your expertise, accomplishments, and industry engagement. Actively participating in relevant professional networks, forums, and discussions positions you as a thought leader, amplifying your influence within your industry.

Strategic content curation is paramount. Sharing insightful articles, thought-provoking commentary, and updates on professional achievements demonstrates your expertise and adds value to your network. The judicious inclusion of personal elements fosters authenticity, humanizing your digital presence and fostering connections beyond the transactional.

Moreover, active engagement in online conversations is a powerful strategy. Responding to comments, participating in discussions, and offering constructive insights not only showcases your knowledge but also builds a community around your brand. Additionally, strategically seeking endorsements and recommendations on platforms like LinkedIn further validates your professional prowess.

A proactive approach to reputation management involves monitoring your online presence, addressing any negative feedback or misconceptions promptly, and showcasing a commitment to continuous learning and improvement. By strategically implementing these online reputation enhancement strategies, professionals in the corporate world can shape a positive and influential digital footprint that aligns with their career goals and contributes to their overall success.

As we navigate the nuances of digital footprint and online presence, remember that the digital realm is not just a passive showcase; it's an active arena where you can shape perceptions, build alliances, and amplify your impact. By leveraging the power of professional networks, finding the right balance in content curation, and implementing effective reputation management strategies, you can transform your online presence into a dynamic force that propels your personal brand to new heights in the interconnected world of work.

Networking: Building Meaningful Connections

In the vast tapestry of professional growth, the art of networking emerges as a thread that weaves together opportunities, insights, and meaningful relationships.

Navigating successful networking events is an art form. Beyond the surface-level engagements, professionals in the corporate world employ strategic introductions, active listening, and purposeful follow-ups to transform fleeting encounters into lasting connections. The ability to navigate these events with finesse is not just a social skill; it's a pathway to building a network that goes beyond the superficial, creating a community of individuals invested in each other's success.

As the digital landscape continues to shape professional interactions, building relationships online becomes an essential aspect of networking. Leveraging platforms like LinkedIn and actively participating in industry forums contribute to the development of a robust virtual network. Beyond self-promotion, the focus is on engaging with the content and contributions of others, creating a reciprocal dynamic that mirrors the depth and authenticity of in-person connections.

In the corporate world, networking is not merely a means to an end; it's a continuous journey of relationship-building that forms the backbone of professional success. By prioritizing quality over quantity, mastering the intricacies of networking events, and seamlessly transitioning these skills into the digital realm, professionals lay the groundwork for a network that not only supports their current endeavors but also opens doors to unforeseen opportunities and collaborations.

Quality over Quantity in Professional Relationships

Networking is not a numbers game; it's about cultivating genuine and impactful connections. This section emphasizes the importance of quality over quantity in building professional relationships. Instead of amassing an extensive but superficial network, the focus shifts to fostering deep, meaningful connections. The strength of your network lies not just in the sheer number of contacts but in the authenticity, trust, and mutual support that characterize each relationship.

Unlike a mere collection of business cards or LinkedIn connections, the emphasis on quality speaks to the depth, authenticity, and enduring value inherent in cultivating genuine professional relationships.

Quality relationships are built on a foundation of trust, shared values, and a genuine understanding of each other's aspirations and challenges. It's not about the sheer volume of contacts but the resonance and impact of each connection. In a world where time is a precious commodity, investing it in building a select few relationships that truly matter yields more significant returns than scattering efforts across a multitude of superficial connections.

The strength of a professional network lies not just in its size but in the reciprocal support, mentorship, and collaboration that characterize the connections within it. Quality relationships provide a robust support system, offering insights, opportunities, and a shared journey toward mutual success. In prioritizing quality over quantity, professionals foster a network that goes beyond the transactional, becoming a community of trusted allies who contribute to each other's growth and prosperity in the dynamic landscape of the professional world.

Chapter Ten

Strategies for Successful Networking Events

Networking events provide fertile ground for cultivating connections, but success in these settings requires a strategic approach. We explore techniques for navigating networking events with confidence, including the art of effective introductions, active listening, and meaningful follow-ups. By mastering these strategies, professionals can transform these events from mere opportunities for small talk into platforms for building lasting connections that transcend the event itself.

Success in these settings requires a multifaceted approach, beginning with the mastery of effective introductions. Crafting an introduction that succinctly communicates who you are and what you bring to the professional table sets the tone for meaningful conversations.

Active listening emerges as a cornerstone strategy. Instead of focusing solely on self-promotion, attentive listening allows you to understand the needs and aspirations of others. This empathetic approach not only forges a genuine connection but also provides a foundation for mutual support and collaboration.

Equally important is the art of meaningful follow-ups. A well-timed and personalized follow-up after a networking event reinforces the connection and demonstrates genuine interest. Whether it's through a personalized email, a LinkedIn message, or a coffee meeting, these follow-ups solidify the initial rapport established during the event.

Additionally, successful networking involves a mindset shift—from viewing these events as opportunities for surface-level interactions to platforms for building long-term relationships. By embracing authenticity, actively engaging with others, and approaching networking events with a genuine curiosity about others' professional journeys, professionals can transform these occasions into pivotal moments for connection, collaboration, and career advancement.

Building Relationships Online

As the digital landscape continues to play a pivotal role in professional interactions, the chapter explores the intricacies of building relationships online. From leveraging professional networks like LinkedIn to participating in industry forums and online communities, we unravel the strategies that transform virtual connections into meaningful relationships. Building relationships online involves not just broadcasting your achievements but actively engaging with the content and contributions of others, fostering a reciprocal dynamic that forms the bedrock of a robust professional network.

In the chapters ahead, we delve deeper into the nuances of networking, understanding that successful networking is not a transaction but a relationship-building journey. By prioritizing quality connections, mastering the art of networking events, and seamlessly transitioning these skills into the digital realm, professionals can cultivate a network that not only supports their current endeavors but also lays the groundwork for future opportunities and collaborations.

Professional Growth Through Thought Leadership

In the ever-evolving landscape of professional growth, the role of thought leadership emerges as a catalyst for individual and collective advancement. Professional growth through thought leadership is a transformative journey of sharing insights, expertise, and innovative ideas to elevate one's influence within an industry. Starting a blog, podcast, or vlog provides a digital canvas to disseminate knowledge and establish authority, creating a valuable repository of content that contributes to an individual's personal brand. By sharing expertise through seminars, webinars, or dynamic presentations, professionals not only position themselves as subject matter experts but also actively contribute to the collective learning of their industry. Collaboration with industry peers further amplifies thought leadership, fostering a culture of shared knowledge and innovation. Thought leadership is not just about personal advancement; it's a strategic and collaborative approach that drives individual and collective growth, positioning professionals as influential voices shaping the future of their fields.

Starting a Blog, Podcast, or Vlog

Thought leadership often begins with the dissemination of knowledge and insights through various mediums. Starting a blog, podcast, or vlog provides a platform to share expertise, perspectives, and industry trends. These digital channels not only position professionals as authoritative voices in their fields but also create a valuable repository of content that contributes to their personal brand. By consistently producing high-quality content, professionals can become go-to resources within their industries.

Starting a blog, podcast, or vlog is a dynamic pathway to professional growth through thought leadership. These platforms transcend traditional boundaries, allowing professionals to amplify their expertise and perspectives to a global audience. By consistently creating valuable content, individuals position themselves as authorities in their respective fields, cultivating a personal brand synonymous with knowledge and innovation. Blogs, with their written format, offer in-depth exploration, while podcasts and vlogs add a personal touch, fostering a deeper connection with the audience. These mediums not only contribute to the individual's growth but also enrich the industry's collective knowledge base. In an era where digital presence is synonymous with influence, starting a blog, podcast, or vlog becomes not just a personal endeavor but a strategic move toward shaping the narrative of one's professional journey and impacting the broader discourse within the industry.

Sharing Expertise via Seminars or Webinars

Seminars and webinars serve as dynamic arenas for thought leadership, offering opportunities to share in-depth knowledge with a targeted audience. Whether it's presenting at industry conferences or hosting webinars on specialized topics, professionals can showcase their expertise while actively engaging with peers and stakeholders. These platforms not only elevate individual profiles but also contribute to the collective learning and growth within the industry.

Sharing expertise via seminars or webinars is a strategic cornerstone of thought leadership, offering professionals a dynamic platform to showcase their knowledge, insights, and innovations. These interactive forums not only elevate individual profiles within their industries but also contribute to the collective learning of the broader professional community. Seminars and webinars provide a direct avenue for professionals to engage with a targeted audience, offering in-depth perspectives on industry trends, best practices, and emerging challenges. By actively participating in these events, thought leaders not only position themselves as authorities in their fields but also foster a culture of continuous learning and knowledge exchange. The impact extends beyond personal growth, influencing the collective intelligence of the industry and establishing a dynamic ecosystem where expertise is shared, challenged, and collectively elevated.

Collaborating with Industry Peers

Collaboration is a cornerstone of thought leadership. By actively engaging with industry peers, professionals can participate in a collective exchange of ideas and insights. Collaborative projects, joint publications, or co-hosted events not only broaden individual networks but also foster a culture of shared expertise. Through strategic collaboration, professionals can leverage collective intelligence to address industry challenges, drive innovation, and position themselves as leaders within a collaborative ecosystem.

Collaborating with industry peers is an indispensable facet of professional growth through thought leadership. In an interconnected world, the exchange of ideas and insights with fellow professionals elevates not only individual profiles but also contributes to the collective intelligence of the industry. By actively participating in collaborative projects, joint publications, or co-hosted events, professionals foster a culture of shared expertise that transcends individual achievements. Such collaborations not only expand individual networks but also create a dynamic ecosystem where knowledge flows seamlessly. The importance lies not just in personal advancement but in the co-creation of innovative solutions, addressing industry challenges collectively, and positioning oneself as a leader within a collaborative community.

Feedback: Using Criticism Constructively

In the continuous journey of professional development, the art of using feedback constructively becomes a transformative force. In the corporate realm, the ability to use feedback constructively is a linchpin for individual and organizational success. Actively seeking feedback is a strategic initiative that propels professionals toward continuous improvement. By actively soliciting insights from colleagues, supervisors, and peers, individuals not only gain a more comprehensive understanding of their strengths and areas for development but also demonstrate a commitment to personal and collective growth.

Filtering and analyzing criticism is an essential skill in navigating the complex landscape of corporate work life. In a fast-paced environment, where decisions are often made swiftly, the capacity to distinguish between subjective opinions and constructive insights is invaluable. It allows professionals to extract actionable elements from feedback, turning criticism into a catalyst for refinement rather than a deterrent.

Actionable steps for continuous improvement transform feedback from a passive evaluation tool into an active driver of progress. By implementing tangible steps based on feedback, professionals enhance their skills, adapt to evolving challenges, and contribute to a culture of excellence within the organization.

Seeking Out Feedback Actively

Proactively seeking feedback is a proactive step toward personal and professional growth. By actively seeking insights from colleagues, mentors, and peers, professionals create a feedback loop that fosters a culture of continuous improvement. Actively seeking feedback not only demonstrates a commitment to growth but also provides valuable perspectives that may not be apparent through self-assessment alone.

Actively seeking feedback in the corporate realm is not merely a professional choice; it's a strategic investment in individual and organizational success. In a dynamic and competitive work environment, the ability to proactively seek insights from colleagues, superiors, and peers is a hallmark of a growth-oriented professional. Actively seeking feedback demonstrates a commitment to continuous improvement and a recognition that growth stems from a willingness to embrace diverse perspectives.

In the corporate context, where collaboration and effective communication are integral, actively seeking feedback becomes a catalyst for enhanced performance. It opens channels for constructive dialogue, encourages a culture of transparency, and fosters stronger working relationships. Professionals who actively seek feedback not only position themselves as adaptable and open to development but also contribute to a workplace culture that values learning and improvement.

Moreover, in the fast-paced corporate landscape, where change is constant, feedback serves as a compass for navigating uncertainties. Actively seeking feedback ensures that professionals remain agile, responsive, and aligned with organizational goals. It transforms the workplace into a dynamic learning environment, where each interaction becomes an opportunity for growth.

Filtering and Analyzing Criticism

Criticism, when filtered and analyzed with a discerning mindset, becomes a powerful tool for growth. This section delves into the art of distinguishing constructive criticism from subjective opinions. Professionals learn to extract valuable insights, identify patterns, and discern actionable elements from the feedback received. By adopting a mindset that views criticism as a catalyst for improvement rather than a deterrent, individuals can leverage feedback to refine their skills and approaches.

Filtering and analyzing criticism is a crucial skill in the pursuit of personal and professional development. Rather than viewing criticism as a mere judgment, it becomes a valuable source of insights and opportunities for growth. The ability to discern between constructive feedback and subjective opinions empowers individuals to extract meaningful lessons from critiques.

Criticism, when filtered with discernment, transforms into a mirror that reflects areas for improvement. It allows professionals to navigate beyond the surface-level comments and identify recurring patterns or themes that may indicate genuine areas for refinement. This discerning approach shifts the narrative from a defensive stance to an open mindset, where feedback is seen as a pathway to mastery rather than a threat.

Moreover, the act of analyzing criticism cultivates resilience and a growth mindset. It encourages individuals to view setbacks not as failures but as stepping stones toward improvement. By understanding the underlying motivations and perspectives behind criticism, professionals can leverage it as a tool for self-awareness, adapting their approaches, and refining their skills.

Actionable Steps for Continuous Improvement

Feedback, when translated into actionable steps, becomes the cornerstone of continuous improvement. This part of the book explores strategies for implementing feedback effectively, transforming insights into tangible actions. Whether it's refining specific skills, adjusting communication styles, or embracing new approaches, professionals learn how to integrate feedback into their ongoing development journey. This iterative process of receiving, analyzing, and acting upon feedback creates a trajectory of continuous improvement, propelling individuals toward their professional best.

The importance of actionable steps for continuous improvement lies in the transformative potential that feedback carries when translated into tangible actions. While feedback provides insights, it is the actionable steps that bridge the gap between awareness and actual growth. By distilling feedback into specific, measurable, and achievable actions, professionals create a roadmap for personal and professional development.

These actionable steps act as the catalyst for change, allowing individuals to address identified areas for improvement with intentionality. Instead of viewing feedback as a mere evaluation, the process of implementing actionable steps transforms it into a dynamic tool for progress. Professionals learn not only to refine existing skills but also to embrace new strategies and approaches that contribute to their ongoing evolution.

Also, the iterative nature of actionable steps fosters a culture of continuous improvement. It's not a one-time fix but a journey of perpetual refinement, where each round of feedback informs the next cycle of growth. By embracing this mindset and integrating actionable steps into their routine, professionals pave the way for sustained excellence, resilience in the face of challenges, and a commitment to lifelong learning and development.

Chapter Eleven

Thriving in Job Interviews

In the intricate dance of job interviews, the skill of thriving extends beyond the mere presentation of qualifications; it's a choreography of preparation, poise, and profound self-awareness. This chapter is your guide to not just surviving but excelling in the critical juncture where careers take shape and destinies are decided.

Understanding the landscape of job interviews is crucial. It's not a mere interrogation; it's a nuanced conversation where your skills, personality, and cultural fit are under scrutiny. Thriving begins with a deep understanding of the company culture, the role you're applying for, and the expectations of the interviewer. Research becomes your ally, offering insights that transform you from a candidate into a strategic fit for the organization.

An interview is your narrative, and you are the storyteller. This chapter delves into the art of crafting a compelling story that seamlessly weaves your experiences, skills, and aspirations into a cohesive narrative. From your introduction to your closing statements, every word is an opportunity to leave a lasting impression. We explore the power of storytelling as a tool for not just conveying information but creating an emotional connection with your interviewer.

Confidence, the recurring theme in our journey, takes center stage in interviews. Thriving is not about showcasing a bravado that masks insecurities; it's about presenting your authentic self with confidence. This chapter delves into the subtleties of body language, tone of voice, and the delicate balance between humility and self-assurance. We uncover the secrets to projecting confidence without crossing into the territory of arrogance.

The questions posed in interviews are not hurdles but stepping stones for you to shine. We navigate the common interview questions, from the classic "Tell me about yourself" to the complex situational inquiries. Thriving in interviews involves more than rehearsing scripted answers; it's about understanding the underlying motivations behind each question and responding with authenticity and relevance. We delve into the STAR method, a structured approach to crafting impactful responses that showcase your skills and accomplishments.

Job interviews are seldom smooth sailing; they often navigate through stormy scenarios such as gaps in your resume, challenging work experiences, or unexpected questions. This chapter equips you with strategies to navigate these challenges with finesse. Thriving involves turning potential weaknesses into strengths, addressing concerns proactively, and maintaining composure in the face of unexpected turns.

The closing moments of an interview are as crucial as the opening ones. Thriving involves leaving a lasting impression, expressing genuine interest, and seeking clarity on the next steps. We explore effective ways to conclude the interview, from asking insightful questions to expressing gratitude for the opportunity. This chapter guides you on how to exit the room not as an interviewee but as a potential colleague and valuable asset.

As you navigate the landscape of job interviews, remember that thriving is not about presenting a flawless facade but about showcasing your authentic self with confidence and competence. Each interview is not just an assessment; it's an opportunity for mutual exploration, where both you and the employer seek the perfect fit. This chapter empowers you to approach interviews not with trepidation but with the confidence of someone who understands their worth and is ready to contribute meaningfully to the professional tapestry. So, step into the interview room not as an outsider seeking approval but as a candidate ready to thrive and contribute to the success of the organization.

Understanding the Interviewer's Mindset

In this pivotal section, we embark on a profound exploration of the intricate nuances that define the interviewer's mindset, unraveling the goals and objectives that form the bedrock of the interview process. This understanding serves not only as a compass but as a strategic advantage, allowing you to align your responses with the core values and mission of the organization.

The first point of our discussion revolves around recognizing the implicit goals and objectives that interviewers harbor. Interviews are not arbitrary interrogations; they are purposeful interactions designed to assess not just your technical skills but also your compatibility with the organization's culture and your potential contributions to its objectives. By peeling back the layers of the interviewer's mindset, you gain insights that transform the interview from a one-sided evaluation into a collaborative exploration of mutual fit.

Addressing implicit biases and making positive first impressions emerge as essential facets of thriving in job interviews. Unconscious biases can subtly influence decisions, making it imperative to navigate these biases with finesse. This section equips you with the tools to preemptively address biases, presenting yourself as a candidate whose qualities transcend preconceived notions. First impressions, often formed within the initial moments of an interview, can significantly impact the interviewer's perception. We delve into the art of crafting a memorable yet authentic introduction, ensuring that your first impression is a testament to your professionalism and suitability for the role.

Soft skills, often the unsung heroes of professional success, take center stage in our exploration. Interviewers seek candidates who not only possess technical prowess but also exhibit interpersonal skills that contribute to a positive and collaborative work environment. Demonstrating these soft skills becomes a strategic move in the interview landscape. From effective communication to adaptability, we unravel the key soft skills that can set you apart and showcase your potential as a valuable team member.

Implicit biases, those unconscious predispositions that color perceptions, are acknowledged as inherent in the human experience. This segment delves into not just recognizing these biases but strategically navigating them. By preemptively addressing potential biases, you position yourself as a candidate who transcends stereotypes, emphasizing your capabilities and potential impact on the organization. It's a dance of self-awareness and strategic communication, where authenticity becomes a powerful tool for dispelling preconceived notions.

Making positive first impressions, often formed within the initial moments of an interview, is an art that goes beyond the confines of a rehearsed introduction. We explore the intricacies of body language, tone, and the subtle cues that communicate professionalism and confidence. This section isn't about crafting a superficial persona but about authentically presenting the best version of yourself—a version that resonates with the interviewer's expectations and leaves a lasting, positive impression.

Cultural fit, a term frequently uttered in hiring discussions, is more than just a buzzword—it's a pivotal factor that determines your compatibility with the organization's values and dynamics. Thriving in interviews involves not only understanding the organization's culture but also articulating how your values align with theirs. We explore strategies to convey cultural fit authentically, ensuring that your presence in the organization contributes positively to its ethos.

As we navigate the intricacies of the interviewer's mindset, remember that this understanding is not a manipulative tool but a strategic guide. It empowers you to present yourself authentically while strategically aligning your responses with the organization's objectives. By recognizing the unspoken goals of interviews, addressing biases, and showcasing soft skills and cultural fit, you transform the interview from a mere evaluation into a collaborative dialogue where both you and the interviewer seek the ideal match.

Preparation: More Than Just Knowing Your Resume

In this section, we embark on a comprehensive exploration of preparation, transcending the boundaries of a mere recitation of your resume. Thriving in job interviews is inseparable from thorough research on the company and the specific role you're applying for. We delve into the nuances of this research, guiding you on how to uncover key information about the company's values, mission, and recent achievements. Understanding the intricacies of the role allows you to tailor your responses to showcase not just your skills but your alignment with the organization's needs.

Anticipating and practicing common questions is a fundamental aspect of preparation. We not only provide an extensive list of commonly asked questions but also guide you on how to structure your responses. Through strategic preparation, you transform these questions into opportunities to highlight your achievements, problem-solving skills, and unique value proposition. This section serves as your toolkit for not just answering questions but crafting responses that leave a lasting impression.

However, thriving in interviews goes beyond being reactive; it involves proactive preparation. We explore the art of preparing unique insights and questions for interviewers. By demonstrating your deep interest in the company and role, you position yourself as an engaged and forward-thinking candidate. This section guides you on how to formulate insightful questions that not only showcase your understanding of the company but also create a dialogue that goes beyond the surface, leaving a memorable impact on the interviewer.

Non-verbal Communication: It's Louder Than Words

This section delves into the profound influence of non-verbal communication, emphasizing that sometimes, it speaks louder than words. We explore the intricate dance of body language and tone, dissecting the subtle messages they convey. From the firmness of a handshake to maintaining eye contact, every non-verbal cue becomes a silent participant in the interview conversation.

The impact of body language and tone extends beyond the realm of conscious awareness. We guide you through the art of using your body language to convey confidence and poise. From the subtle cues of open posture to the intentional modulation of your voice, each element contributes to the overall impression you leave on the interviewer. Understanding and harnessing this silent language becomes a powerful tool for not just expressing but embodying confidence.

However, mastering non-verbal communication is a nuanced skill that involves more than adopting a set of prescribed gestures. This section provides concrete strategies for conveying confidence authentically. It's not about putting on a performance but about aligning your non-verbal cues with your genuine feelings of self-assurance. We explore techniques that allow you to navigate the delicate balance between projecting confidence and maintaining authenticity.

Navigating the delicate terrain of an interview demands more than just the right words—it requires a symphony of strategies to convey confidence and poise. In this intricate dance, we delve into the art of strategic non-verbal communication, offering a nuanced understanding of how to authentically project assurance.

One key strategy is mastering the power of eye contact. Sustained and purposeful eye contact communicates attentiveness, sincerity, and self-assurance. We explore techniques that go beyond mere staring, guiding you on how to maintain eye contact naturally and comfortably. The eyes, often described as windows to the soul, become a powerful instrument for expressing your confidence without uttering a word.

Another essential strategy involves the intentional use of gestures. From the firmness of your handshake to the subtlety of your hand movements, gestures can either enhance or detract from your message. This section provides actionable insights into using gestures to underscore your points, creating a visual rhythm that complements your verbal communication. It's about striking the right balance—using gestures to amplify your words without overshadowing them.

Posture, often an overlooked aspect of non-verbal communication, emerges as a strategic tool for conveying confidence and poise. We explore the nuances of open and closed postures, guiding you on how to use your body language to project confidence. From sitting up straight to maintaining an open and engaged stance, each posture cue becomes a brushstroke in the canvas of your non-verbal narrative.

Moreover, the strategic modulation of your tone of voice becomes a powerful element in conveying confidence. We delve into the art of speaking with clarity, using a measured pace, and inflecting your voice to emphasize key points. By mastering the subtle dynamics of tone, you not only express confidence but also captivate your audience, creating an engaging and compelling presence.

These strategies are not about adopting a rehearsed set of behaviors but about enhancing your natural presence. It's about aligning your non-verbal cues with your authentic self, ensuring that every gesture, every glance, and every intonation reflects the confidence that resides within. By incorporating these strategies into your non-verbal repertoire, you elevate your interview performance from a mere exchange of information to a captivating and memorable conversation.

Avoiding common non-verbal mistakes becomes a crucial aspect of this exploration. From fidgeting to avoiding eye contact, subtle errors can undermine the impact of your verbal communication. We dissect these common pitfalls and provide actionable tips on how to sidestep them. The goal is not to create a rigid set of rules but to enhance your awareness of your non-verbal cues, ensuring that they complement your verbal responses rather than detract from them.

It can be said that non-verbal communication becomes an art form that, when mastered, enhances your overall interview performance. By understanding the impact of body language and tone, strategically conveying confidence and poise, and avoiding common non-verbal mistakes, you transform your silent language into a symphony that harmonizes with your verbal expressions, creating a cohesive and compelling narrative in the interview room.

Handling Tricky Questions and Scenarios

In this critical section, we navigate the challenging terrain of tricky questions and scenarios, equipping you with the skills to address them with finesse and confidence. The first point of focus is addressing gaps in employment or tricky situations. We delve into strategies that transform these potential stumbling blocks into stepping stones, emphasizing transparency, growth, and the lessons learned during these periods.

Turning perceived weaknesses into strengths becomes an essential aspect of thriving in interviews. Rather than shying away from vulnerabilities, we explore the art of reframing them as opportunities for growth and development. This section provides actionable insights on how to communicate your awareness of weaknesses while showcasing your proactive approach to overcoming them. It's a strategic move that transforms challenges into narratives of resilience and continuous improvement.

Staying calm and composed under pressure is a skill that sets apart thriving candidates. Interviews, especially when confronted with tricky questions or unexpected scenarios, can be high-pressure situations. We delve into techniques for maintaining your composure, from controlled breathing to strategic pauses. By mastering the art of staying centered, you not only convey confidence but also demonstrate your ability to think critically and navigate challenges with grace.

In the dynamic landscape of the corporate world, the ability to stay calm and composed under pressure emerges as a hallmark of effective leadership and professionalism. This skill is not just a personal asset but a strategic advantage that can influence decision-making, team dynamics, and overall performance.

Corporate environments are rife with situations that demand a cool and collected demeanor—be it during high-stakes meetings, tight deadlines, or unexpected challenges. Executives and leaders who can navigate these pressure-cooker scenarios with grace become beacons of stability in the turbulent seas of corporate life. It's not about eliminating stress but about managing it in a way that doesn't compromise your judgment or communication.

One key aspect of staying calm under pressure is maintaining a strategic perspective. In the face of tight deadlines or challenging projects, the ability to step back, assess the situation objectively, and prioritize tasks becomes invaluable. This strategic mindset not only aids in decision-making but also inspires confidence in your leadership, reassuring team members that challenges are being addressed with a thoughtful approach.

Moreover, effective communication is amplified when delivered with calmness. In high-pressure situations, the corporate world values leaders who can convey messages clearly and confidently. The ability to articulate plans, updates, or solutions in a composed manner not only fosters a sense of assurance but also inspires trust among colleagues, clients, and stakeholders.

Staying calm under pressure is not a static trait but a skill that can be cultivated through practice and self-awareness. Techniques such as mindfulness, time management, and adaptive thinking contribute to a resilient mindset. Corporate leaders who invest in honing this skill not only enhance their individual performance but also contribute to a positive and resilient organizational culture.

It is obvious that the corporate world is a crucible where pressure refines leadership. Those who can remain calm and composed in the face of adversity not only navigate challenges effectively but also inspire confidence in their ability to steer the ship through turbulent waters. As we explore strategies for staying calm under pressure in interviews, it's essential to recognize that this skill transcends the confines of a single interaction—it's a cornerstone of success in the corporate arena, where the ability to thrive amidst challenges is not just an asset but a testament to true leadership.

This section serves as a guide for not just surviving but excelling when faced with the unpredictable twists and turns of interviews. By addressing gaps in employment with transparency, turning perceived weaknesses into narratives of growth, and staying calm under pressure, you transform tricky questions and scenarios into opportunities to showcase your resilience, adaptability, and unwavering confidence.

Follow-up and Feedback

In this concluding section, we shift our focus to the often underestimated yet pivotal phases of follow-up and feedback. Crafting a memorable thank-you note emerges as a strategic move that extends beyond mere courtesy. We delve into the art of expressing gratitude while reiterating your enthusiasm for the role. This section provides insights on how to personalize your thank-you note, making it a memorable and impactful addition to your post-interview communication.

Seeking feedback post-rejection is a powerful tool for continuous improvement. Rather than viewing rejection as a closed chapter, we explore the proactive approach of seeking feedback. This section guides you on how to reach out to interviewers, asking for constructive insights that can inform your future endeavors. The ability to turn rejection into a learning opportunity not only fosters personal growth but positions you as a candidate committed to continuous development.

Continual learning and preparation for future opportunities form the cornerstone of this final point. Thriving in the professional world is not a destination but a journey of perpetual evolution. We discuss strategies for ongoing learning, whether through courses, workshops, or staying abreast of industry trends. The proactive mindset of preparing for future opportunities, even after a rejection, becomes a testament to your resilience and commitment to professional growth.

In the corporate world, the ability to transform rejection into a catalyst for growth is a skill that distinguishes resilient and proactive professionals. Seeking feedback post-rejection is not just a gesture; it's a strategic move that reflects a commitment to continuous improvement and a nuanced understanding of the value of constructive insights.

In the face of rejection, the initial emotional response might be disappointment or frustration. However, the seasoned professional understands that beyond the closed door of an opportunity lies a pathway to self-discovery and enhancement. Seeking feedback post-rejection is an embodiment of this mindset—a recognition that every setback is a classroom, and every rejection is a lesson waiting to be learned.

Approaching interviewers or hiring managers for feedback requires a delicate balance of humility and curiosity. It's not about challenging the decision but about understanding the nuances that influenced it. Professionals who can navigate this process with grace position themselves as candidates who are not just seeking validation but are genuinely invested in their professional development.

The feedback obtained post-rejection serves as a roadmap for improvement. It might highlight areas where your skills align perfectly and areas that could benefit from enhancement. It's an opportunity to gain insights into the expectations of the corporate environment and to understand how you can better align your skills and presentation with those expectations.

Moreover, the act of seeking feedback post-rejection communicates resilience and a growth mindset. It sends a powerful message that you view setbacks not as roadblocks but as stepping stones. This proactive approach doesn't go unnoticed in the corporate world, where the ability to bounce back from challenges is highly valued.

As we navigate the realms of follow-up and feedback, remember that these phases are not mere formalities but strategic moves in the chessboard of your professional journey. Crafting a memorable thank-you note, seeking feedback post-rejection, and committing to continual learning create a narrative of persistence, self-awareness, and a genuine passion for professional development. Through these actions, you not only leave a lasting impression on the interviewers but also position yourself as a candidate who views every experience as a stepping stone toward future success.

Chapter Twelve

Navigating Career Changes and Transitions

This chapter takes you on a journey through the intricate landscape of career changes and transitions. In this ever-evolving professional realm, change is not a mere possibility but a constant. This chapter serves as your guide to not only navigate through these transitions but to thrive in the face of them.

The narrative begins by challenging the conventional notion of a linear career path. It encourages you to see change not as a threat but as an opportunity for growth and reinvention. Through real-world examples, the chapter illustrates how professionals who embrace change often find themselves on an accelerated path to success. The ability to pivot, view change as a chance for skill enhancement, and leverage past experiences become a distinguishing feature of a confident and agile professional.

Navigating a career transition requires more than a polished resume. It demands a strategic mindset, resilience to handle uncertainties, and a roadmap for personal and professional reinvention. This chapter introduces a toolkit of strategies, from effective networking in a new industry to upskilling for a career shift. It delves into the psychology of change, addressing the fears and uncertainties that often accompany a transition. By understanding the emotional landscape of change, professionals can develop the mental fortitude to weather challenges and emerge stronger.

In a world where personal branding is as crucial as professional qualifications, this chapter guides you through the process of building a personal brand that transcends industries. It explores the importance of a consistent online presence, the art of storytelling in interviews, and the strategic use of transferable skills to position yourself as an asset in any professional setting. Recognizing that a career transition is about aligning your professional narrative with evolving goals, the chapter offers exercises and reflections to articulate your unique value proposition.

Successful career transitions are often fueled by meaningful connections. This chapter offers practical insights into networking strategies, emphasizing the importance of authenticity and reciprocity in building a robust professional network. Additionally, it explores the role of mentors in guiding you through transitions, providing not just advice but a roadmap drawn from their own experiences.

No career transition is without its challenges. This chapter prepares you for the inevitable setbacks, offering tools to bounce back with resilience. It's not just about weathering the storm but learning to dance in the rain, understanding that setbacks are not roadblocks but detours leading to unexpected opportunities.

As you navigate the intricate terrain of career changes, this chapter is your companion, offering not just guidance but a mindset shift. Career transitions are not interruptions to your journey; they are the threads weaving the rich tapestry of your professional story. By approaching change with confidence and adaptability, you transform what could be perceived as obstacles into stepping stones toward a more fulfilling and dynamic career.

Recognizing When It's Time to Move On

In the complex dance of a career, recognizing the right moment to step onto a new stage is a skill that goes beyond the black and white of job descriptions. This section dives into the nuances of recognizing the signs that whisper, and sometimes shout, that it's time for a change. The traditional notion of a lifelong commitment to a single company or role has evolved into a more fluid and responsive approach to career management.

Job satisfaction, often regarded as the cornerstone of professional contentment, holds the power to shape the trajectory of an individual's career. When an individual is attuned to the signals of diminishing job satisfaction, it serves as an early warning system, signaling that the alignment between personal values, work responsibilities, and organizational culture might be unraveling.

Equally crucial is the assessment of growth potential within a current role. In a corporate ecosystem that thrives on innovation and adaptability, professionals are akin to dynamic entities, continually evolving and seeking new challenges. Recognizing when your current position no longer provides the necessary platform for growth and skill development empowers you to make strategic decisions that align with your long-term aspirations.

Understanding personal and professional goals is a compass that guides career decisions. The corporate journey is not merely a series of job titles but a path toward the fulfillment of personal and professional objectives. When there is a misalignment between your current role and these goals, it's a pivotal moment to consider a shift, realigning your career trajectory with your authentic aspirations.

Emotional and mental well-being, often overlooked in traditional career discourse, plays a paramount role in recognizing the need for change. The toll of persisting in a role that no longer brings joy or purpose can manifest in burnout, frustration, or a sense of stagnation. Acknowledging these emotional and mental signs becomes a form of self-care, signaling the importance of prioritizing one's well-being in the professional journey.

Analyzing Job Satisfaction and Growth Potential

Job satisfaction is the heartbeat of a fulfilling career. We'll explore how to conduct a thorough self-assessment, examining the aspects of your current role that bring joy, fulfillment, and a sense of purpose. Simultaneously, we delve into growth potential—evaluating whether your current position aligns with your aspirations and offers the room for professional development.

Job satisfaction serves as the pulse, the rhythmic beat that reverberates through every professional endeavor. It encapsulates not just the tasks on your to-do list but the intrinsic joy derived from the work you engage in daily. A satisfying job isn't merely a checkbox; it's the cornerstone of a fulfilling career, where passion and purpose converge.

Equally paramount is the exploration of growth potential within the corporate landscape. In a dynamic environment where change is constant, a career that fosters continuous development is a career that thrives. The corporate world is a bustling marketplace of skills, where staying relevant is as crucial as acquiring competence. Assessing the growth potential of your current role involves scrutinizing not only the opportunities for advancement but also the avenues for skill enhancement and professional evolution. It's about envisioning your trajectory not as a static line but as an upward spiral, where each step propels you toward greater competence, leadership, and accomplishment.

Understanding Personal and Professional Goals

Aligning your career with your personal and professional goals is key to sustained fulfillment. This section prompts reflection on your long-term objectives and how well your current role propels you toward them. By understanding the synergy between your aspirations and your career trajectory, you gain clarity on when a change is not just beneficial but necessary.

Understanding personal and professional goals in the corporate world is akin to having a well-calibrated compass on a challenging expedition. It's not just about reaching a destination; it's about aligning your journey with your innermost aspirations. In the dynamic landscape of corporate endeavors, clarity on personal and professional goals serves as the guiding force that propels individuals toward sustained fulfillment and success.

Professionally, having a clear understanding of your goals transforms the abstract concept of success into tangible milestones. It directs your focus, allowing you to make strategic decisions that align with your aspirations. Whether it's choosing a particular career trajectory, pursuing additional qualifications, or seeking leadership roles, the clarity derived from personal and professional goal-setting becomes the lens through which you evaluate opportunities and make informed choices.

Emotional and Mental Signs of Necessary Change

The importance of recognizing emotional and mental signs as indicators for necessary change cannot be overstated in the context of a career transition. While job satisfaction and growth potential are measurable metrics, the emotional and mental well-being of an individual is the pulse that reflects the deeper, often unspoken, aspects of professional life.

Emotional signs, such as a persistent sense of dissatisfaction, a lack of enthusiasm, or feelings of being undervalued, serve as whispers from the inner self. Ignoring these whispers may lead to a gradual erosion of passion and commitment, affecting not only professional performance but also personal well-being.

Mental signs, on the other hand, can manifest as burnout, fatigue, or a sense of disconnection. These are red flags signaling that the current career path may be incongruent with one's authentic self and aspirations. Acknowledging these mental cues is an act of self-compassion, recognizing that mental health is a cornerstone of overall well-being.

In a world where professional success is often equated with external achievements, this section underscores the profound truth that emotional and mental alignment is the bedrock of sustained happiness and success. By tuning into these internal signals, individuals empower themselves to make informed decisions, steering their careers toward paths that resonate with their truest selves.

Beyond the metrics and performance reviews, your emotions and mental well-being are crucial indicators. We discuss the emotional toll of staying in a role that no longer serves you, exploring signs of burnout, frustration, or a sense of stagnation. Recognizing these emotional and mental cues becomes the compass guiding you towards a career path that aligns with your authentic self.

Chapter Thirteen

Achieving Work-Life Balance in a Demanding World

In the relentless pursuit of professional success, the elusive concept of work-life balance often becomes a casualty. Chapter 7 invites you to step off the corporate treadmill and explore the delicate art of harmonizing career ambitions with personal well-being.

The modern professional landscape, with its 24/7 connectivity and ever-increasing demands, has blurred the lines between the office and home. Achieving a work-life balance is not about dividing your time in half but rather about integrating the various facets of your life in a way that nurtures both professional growth and personal fulfillment.

Let's begin by dispelling a common myth—the notion that work-life balance is a static state to be achieved. In reality, it's a dynamic equilibrium that requires constant adjustments. It's about recognizing the ebb and flow of priorities, acknowledging that there will be seasons of intense professional focus and others where personal life takes the spotlight.

A crucial aspect of this chapter is understanding that work-life balance is a personal journey. What works for one person may not work for another. It's about aligning your choices with your values and priorities. This chapter provides practical strategies to help you assess your unique circumstances, identify your priorities, and create a roadmap that integrates both your professional and personal aspirations.

The chapter delves into the role of boundaries—setting them, respecting them, and renegotiating them when necessary. Establishing clear boundaries between work and personal life is not a sign of weakness but a declaration of self-respect. It's about communicating your limits to colleagues, superiors, and even yourself, fostering an environment where personal time is valued as much as professional achievements.

We explore the concept of mindfulness as a powerful tool in achieving work-life balance. Mindfulness is not just about meditation; it's a mindset—an awareness of the present moment that allows you to savor the joys of personal life without the looming shadow of professional stress. The chapter introduces practical exercises and techniques to cultivate mindfulness amidst the chaos of a demanding career.

Moreover, achieving work-life balance is intrinsically linked to effective time management. The chapter offers strategies to prioritize tasks, delegate responsibilities, and make the most of your productive hours. It's not about working longer but working smarter, ensuring that your professional endeavors leave room for personal experiences that bring joy and fulfillment.

In addressing the demanding world we navigate, the chapter acknowledges the role of technology and its impact on work-life integration. While technology enables flexibility, it also poses the risk of constant connectivity. This chapter provides insights into leveraging technology to your advantage, creating digital boundaries, and embracing the tools that enhance efficiency without sacrificing personal time.

A significant portion of the chapter is dedicated to the importance of self-care. The modern professional often neglects their well-being in the pursuit of success. We explore the concept of self-care as a non-negotiable aspect of work-life balance—nourishing your physical, mental, and emotional health to ensure sustained professional excellence.

As we conclude the chapter, the emphasis is on the holistic nature of work-life balance. It's not a checklist but a mindset that recognizes the interconnectedness of professional and personal fulfillment. The chapter provides a roadmap for crafting a life where success is not measured solely by career milestones but by the richness of personal experiences and relationships.

Rethinking the Myth of "Having It All"

In a world that often defines success by the sheer magnitude of professional accomplishments, it's essential to redefine our understanding of fulfillment. This section invites readers to reconsider the myth of "having it all" by exploring the evolving definition of success. We delve into the notion that success is not a one-size-fits-all concept but a dynamic, individualized journey.

In the corporate world, the conventional notion of "having it all" has undergone a profound transformation. The traditional narrative, which once equated success solely with relentless professional ascent, is evolving. The modern professional is challenged to redefine success, recognizing that it extends beyond corner offices and hierarchical climbs.

"Rethinking the Myth of 'Having It All' in the Corporate World" urges professionals to break free from the constraints of a uniform definition of success. It illuminates the changing corporate landscape where success is no longer a monolithic pinnacle but a dynamic spectrum encompassing personal fulfillment, professional achievements, and meaningful relationships.

This paradigm shift encourages individuals to discern their unique priorities within the corporate context. It emphasizes the importance of aligning personal values with professional pursuits, acknowledging that success isn't a zero-sum game. Rather, it's about navigating the complexities of the corporate world while nurturing personal aspirations and relationships.

Ultimately, in this corporate renaissance, professionals are empowered to craft a narrative where success is a harmonious blend of career milestones and personal contentment. The myth of "having it all" transforms from an elusive ideal into a tangible, individualized journey within the corporate tapestry.

The Changing Definition of Success

We navigate the cultural shifts and changing paradigms that have transformed the traditional definition of success. From climbing the corporate ladder to embracing a holistic approach, success is explored as a multifaceted gem, with each facet reflecting personal, professional, and relational achievements.

Once confined to traditional metrics such as hierarchical advancement and financial achievements, success is now recognized as a nuanced and multifaceted concept. The contemporary professional sphere acknowledges that climbing the corporate ladder is just one facet of a much richer tapestry.

Success in the corporate realm has evolved beyond mere job titles and corner offices. It encompasses a holistic approach that embraces qualities like adaptability, innovation, and a commitment to continuous learning. Professionals are increasingly valued not just for their technical prowess but for their ability to navigate change, foster collaboration, and contribute to a positive organizational culture.

Furthermore, the changing definition of success reflects a broader societal shift toward a more inclusive and diverse workforce. Success is not solely measured by individual accomplishments but also by the collective achievements of teams and organizations. The modern corporate paradigm celebrates leadership styles that prioritize empathy, emotional intelligence, and a genuine commitment to the well-being of employees.

Recognizing Individual Priorities

Work-life balance is inherently personal, shaped by individual values and priorities. This point emphasizes the importance of self-reflection to identify and prioritize aspects of life that hold the utmost significance. By recognizing individual priorities, professionals can align their efforts with what truly matters to them.

Balancing Personal and Professional Aspirations: The section offers strategies for striking a delicate balance between personal and professional aspirations. It's not about choosing one over the other but finding the equilibrium that allows for the pursuit of professional goals without sacrificing the richness of personal experiences.

It involves a conscious examination of what holds intrinsic value for an individual amidst the myriad expectations of the professional arena. This process begins with introspection, where professionals identify their core values, personal goals, and the aspects of life that bring them genuine fulfillment.

Individual priorities in the corporate context encompass a spectrum of factors—ranging from career ambitions and professional growth to maintaining a healthy work-life balance. It involves acknowledging that success is not a monolithic construct but a mosaic of achievements tailored to one's unique aspirations. For some, climbing the corporate ladder might be a priority, while for others, meaningful relationships, personal development, or contributing to a larger societal purpose may take precedence.

Recognizing individual priorities empowers professionals to align their efforts with what truly matters to them, fostering a sense of purpose and fulfillment. It encourages authenticity in goal-setting and decision-making, ultimately leading to a more harmonious integration of personal and professional pursuits in the complex tapestry of the corporate world.

By unraveling the myth of "having it all," this section of the book serves as a foundation for readers to embark on a journey of intentional living, where success is not measured by external standards but by the alignment of one's choices with their unique values and aspirations.

Setting Boundaries for Personal Well-being

In the relentless pace of the professional world, the concept of setting boundaries emerges as a crucial cornerstone for safeguarding personal well-being. This section delves into the importance of downtime and mental health, emphasizing that just as professional endeavors demand attention, so does the intricate landscape of your inner world.

The relentless pursuit of professional success often blurs the lines between work and personal life, creating a scenario where individuals find themselves on a perpetual treadmill, with little room for respite.

In this context, establishing boundaries becomes a strategic imperative rather than a mere personal preference. The corporate landscape is inherently demanding, and without intentional efforts to delineate personal time and professional commitments, the risk of burnout looms large. The toll on mental health is undeniable—stress, anxiety and a sense of perpetual urgency can erode both individual well-being and overall productivity.

Setting boundaries in the corporate world is not a sign of weakness; rather, it is an assertion of self-respect and an acknowledgment of the holistic nature of success. It's about creating a sustainable framework that allows individuals to bring their best selves to the professional arena without sacrificing their personal lives. By fostering a culture that values and supports the establishment of clear boundaries, corporations not only enhance the well-being of their employees but also cultivate a resilient workforce capable of navigating challenges with clarity, focus, and sustained excellence.

Importance of Downtime and Mental Health

Work-life balance begins with acknowledging the paramount importance of downtime and mental health. In a culture that often glorifies busyness, this section explores the essential role that moments of rest and rejuvenation play in sustaining long-term professional excellence. It's not merely about physical rest; it's about nurturing your mental and emotional reservoirs, and recognizing that a healthy mind is the bedrock of professional success.

Downtime serves as the essential interval where the mind decompresses, recalibrates, and rejuvenates. It is during these intervals of rest that creativity sparks, problem-solving skills sharpen, and overall cognitive function optimizes. The corporate landscape, with its relentless demands and ever-evolving challenges, places an immense cognitive load on professionals. Without the sanctuary of downtime, the mind becomes susceptible to burnout, fatigue, and diminished productivity.

Furthermore, mental health is not a luxury but a fundamental aspect of an individual's ability to navigate the complexities of the professional world. Stress, anxiety, and exhaustion are not mere inconveniences but formidable adversaries that, if left unaddressed, can jeopardize both personal well-being and professional efficacy. By recognizing the importance of mental health, corporations foster an environment that not only values the holistic well-being of their employees but also unlocks the full spectrum of their creative and innovative potential. In embracing downtime and prioritizing mental health, the corporate world not only safeguards the welfare of its workforce but also cultivates a culture that thrives on the symbiosis of personal and professional flourishing.

Techniques to Disconnect from Work

Building on the premise that personal well-being necessitates intentional disconnection from work, this part provides a toolbox of practical techniques. From mindful disengagement rituals to strategic time management, you'll discover actionable strategies to create a clear demarcation between the professional and personal spheres. These techniques are designed not just to prevent burnout but to cultivate a mindset that cherishes and protects your personal time.

The significance of these techniques lies in their power to safeguard mental and emotional well-being. In a world where the boundary between office and home is often blurred by digital devices, intentional disengagement becomes a counterbalance to prevent burnout and cultivate resilience. By implementing these techniques, professionals can create a sacred space for personal time, allowing the mind to recharge and rejuvenate.

Building a Supportive Ecosystem at Home and Work

Recognizing that setting boundaries is a collaborative effort, this section explores the crucial role of a supportive ecosystem. It's not just about personal boundaries but also about fostering an environment, both at home and work, that values and respects the need for work-life harmony. From open communication with family members to establishing workplace policies that prioritize well-being, building a supportive ecosystem becomes a shared responsibility that amplifies the effectiveness of individual boundary-setting efforts.

In the workplace, cultivating a supportive ecosystem is equally critical. It involves the establishment of policies and cultural norms that prioritize employee well-being. This can manifest in flexible work arrangements, recognition of personal boundaries, and a leadership ethos that values the holistic development of its team members. A supportive work environment not only enhances individual work-life balance but also contributes to increased job satisfaction, productivity, and overall organizational success. Ultimately, building a supportive ecosystem transforms the pursuit of work-life balance from an individual endeavor to a shared commitment, creating a space where both personal and professional aspirations can flourish in tandem.

Time Management and Productivity Hacks

In the intricate dance of work and life, mastering the orchestration of time becomes a pivotal skill. This section serves as your compass in the realm of time management and productivity, guiding you through effective techniques, essential tools, and the transformative power of delegation and trust.

In the professional sphere, effective time management translates to increased efficiency, reduced stress, and a heightened ability to meet deadlines. It allows individuals to navigate through a myriad of tasks without succumbing to being overwhelmed, fostering a sense of accomplishment and boosting overall job satisfaction. Productivity hacks, ranging from focused work intervals to leveraging technological tools, amplified output, transforming work from a mere routine to a dynamic, purposeful endeavor.

Beyond the workplace, mastering time management is a gateway to achieving work-life balance. By optimizing the use of time, individuals carve out space for personal pursuits, family, and self-care. Productivity hacks become the bridge between aspirations and accomplishments, ensuring that personal and professional spheres not only coexist but synergize, creating a life where each moment aligns with one's broader objectives.

Effective Techniques to Manage One's Day

At the heart of work-life balance lies the ability to navigate the hours of your day with purpose and precision. We unravel a spectrum of effective techniques, tailored to accommodate diverse work styles and preferences. Dive into the Pomodoro Technique, a rhythmic dance between focused work and rejuvenating breaks, optimizing your cognitive resources. Explore the Eisenhower Matrix, a strategic framework that empowers you to categorize tasks based on urgency and importance, offering a roadmap to prioritize with clarity. Learn the art of setting realistic goals, breaking down monumental tasks into manageable milestones, and crafting a daily routine that seamlessly aligns with both your professional ambitions and personal dreams.

Tools and Software to Enhance Productivity

In the digital age, an array of productivity tools and software stand ready to amplify your efficiency. Navigate this expansive landscape with our insightful guide, exploring tools that transcend mere convenience and become integral to your daily workflow. Immerse yourself in project management platforms that foster seamless collaboration among team members, transcending geographical constraints. Uncover time-tracking apps that not only account for every minute but also unveil patterns, allowing you to reclaim control over your schedule. We navigate the delicate balance of leveraging technology without succumbing to information overload, ensuring that these digital allies enhance rather than overwhelm your productivity.

Importance of Delegation and Trust

Delegation, often underestimated, emerges as a cornerstone in the architecture of work-life equilibrium. Delve into the intricacies of effective delegation, transcending the mere assignment of tasks to the empowerment of your team. Understand that delegation is not just about offloading responsibilities but fostering a culture of trust within your professional ecosystem. We explore the psychological nuances, dissecting the fear and reluctance associated with relinquishing control. Discover how strategic delegation allows you to elevate your focus to high-impact activities, liberating mental bandwidth for personal priorities. In this exploration, delegation transforms from a managerial tactic to a transformative strategy, reshaping the dynamics of your professional landscape.

This section isn't just a theoretical exploration of time management; it's a practical toolkit, equipping you with the skills, insights, and tools needed to reclaim your time. Work and life need not exist in opposition; they can harmonize when guided by the principles of effective time management, strategic tool usage, and the artful dance of delegation and trust. Welcome to a realm where productivity is not a relentless taskmaster but a reliable ally in your pursuit of a balanced and fulfilling life.

Stress Management and Coping Strategies

In the relentless pursuit of professional success, the shadow of stress often looms large. In the arena of the corporate world, stress management and coping strategies are not merely suggested practices; they are essential survival tools. Recognizing the signs of burnout becomes a critical skill for professionals navigating the relentless demands of their careers. The corporate landscape, characterized by tight deadlines, heavy workloads, and constant connectivity, often becomes a breeding ground for stress. Identifying symptoms such as chronic fatigue, decreased productivity, and emotional exhaustion becomes paramount for individuals to intervene before reaching a state of burnout.

The corporate world demands a proactive approach to stress management. In this context, activities and routines designed to de-stress take center stage. From mindfulness practices that promote mental clarity to engaging in hobbies that provide a therapeutic escape, professionals need a diverse toolkit to navigate the pressures of the workplace. Importantly, these activities are not viewed as indulgences but as strategic investments in maintaining optimal performance and well-being.

Moreover, the corporate culture plays a pivotal role in shaping stress management strategies. Organizations that prioritize employee well-being through flexible work arrangements, wellness programs, and a supportive environment contribute significantly to stress reduction. In the corporate world, seeking professional help is not a sign of weakness but a savvy acknowledgment of the challenges posed by the demanding professional landscape. Ultimately, stress management and coping strategies are integral components of a successful and sustainable career in the corporate world.

Recognizing Signs of Burnout

The chapter opens with a candid discussion of the subtle and not-so-subtle signs of burnout. It's a reality that modern professionals face increasing pressure and expectations, often leading to chronic stress that manifests in physical, emotional, and behavioral symptoms. From persistent fatigue and cynicism to a diminishing sense of accomplishment, recognizing these signs becomes the first step toward effective stress management.

In the corporate world, recognizing signs of burnout is paramount as professionals navigate the demanding landscape. Subtle cues often whisper the impending threat of burnout—persistent fatigue despite adequate rest, a pervasive sense of cynicism towards work, and a diminishing feeling of accomplishment in tasks once found fulfilling. These signs manifest as a result of prolonged exposure to chronic stressors, a common occurrence in high-pressure corporate environments.

The corporate culture's relentless pace, coupled with the ever-present drive for achievement, can blind individuals to the gradual erosion of their well-being. A critical aspect of recognizing burnout is acknowledging the toll unrelenting work demands can take on mental and emotional health. This includes a heightened sensitivity to workplace dynamics, changes in interpersonal relationships, and a decline in overall job satisfaction.

By fostering awareness of these signs, professionals gain a proactive edge against burnout, enabling them to intervene before reaching a state of exhaustion. This self-awareness becomes a powerful tool in the arsenal against burnout, fostering a workplace culture where mental health is prioritized, and individuals are empowered to seek the necessary support and make informed decisions to protect their overall well-being.

Activities and Routines to De-Stress:

Building on the foundation of recognition, the chapter unfolds a comprehensive toolkit of activities and routines designed to alleviate stress and prevent burnout. From mindfulness practices such as meditation and deep breathing exercises to the therapeutic benefits of hobbies and physical activity, the chapter offers a diverse range of strategies tailored to different preferences and lifestyles.

The discussion emphasizes the importance of incorporating these stress-relief activities into daily and weekly routines. They are not mere indulgences but essential components of a holistic approach to well-being. The chapter guides readers in creating a personalized de-stressing plan, encouraging experimentation to identify the activities that resonate most effectively with individual needs.

Additionally, the section addresses the role of a supportive work environment in facilitating stress management. From flexible work arrangements to wellness programs, the modern workplace has the potential to be a partner in promoting employee well-being. Through actionable tips and insights, the chapter guides professionals in navigating workplace dynamics to create a conducive environment for stress reduction.

Seeking Professional Help When Necessary

The stigma surrounding mental health issues in the workplace is dismantled, and the chapter encourages open conversations about well-being.

Readers are guided on how to recognize when stress has transitioned into a more serious mental health concern and are equipped with information on the available resources. Whether it's through employee assistance programs, counseling services, or external mental health professionals, the chapter emphasizes that seeking help is not a sign of weakness but a proactive step toward recovery and resilience.

Pursuing Hobbies and Passions Outside Work

In the perpetual hustle of the professional sphere, where the demands of work often blur into the contours of personal life, the quest for work-life balance becomes a nuanced dance. The pursuit of hobbies and passions outside of work is a profound journey of self-discovery and holistic well-being. Engaging in activities that bring joy and fulfillment contributes not only to personal happiness but also enhances overall life satisfaction. Hobbies serve as an antidote to the stresses of the professional world, offering a therapeutic escape into realms of creativity, self-expression, and relaxation. They provide a crucial counterbalance to the demands of the workplace, fostering resilience and emotional well-being.

Moreover, the significance of pursuing hobbies lies in their ability to shape one's identity beyond the constraints of job titles and responsibilities. Hobbies are threads in the intricate tapestry of individuality, reminding us that our worth extends beyond professional achievements. They cultivate a sense of purpose, allowing individuals to explore and celebrate dimensions of themselves that may be overlooked in the relentless pursuit of career success.

Rediscovering Old Hobbies or Exploring New Ones

In the tapestry of our lives, hobbies are the threads that weave together moments of joy, creativity, and self-expression. They are the fragments of our identity that often get overshadowed by the pressing demands of the professional world. Rediscovering old hobbies is akin to tracing back one's footsteps, navigating through the corridors of nostalgia, and rekindling the flames of past passions.

Perhaps it's the musical instrument gathering dust in the corner, the neglected canvas awaiting the touch of a brush, or the unread novels lining the shelves. Rediscovering these forgotten pursuits is not just a journey into the past but a reconnection with the essence of self—a retrieval of passions that have, in the course of professional pursuits, momentarily slipped into the background.

Simultaneously, there's an invitation to explore the uncharted territories of new hobbies. Novelty, after all, is a catalyst for growth and rejuvenation. Venturing into activities one has never tried becomes a celebration of curiosity and a declaration that personal evolution knows no bounds. The blank canvas of a new hobby holds the promise of unexplored dimensions of oneself waiting to be uncovered.

The Role of Hobbies in Personal Fulfillment

Hobbies are more than mere pastimes; they are portals to personal fulfillment. Within the strokes of a paintbrush, the notes of a musical composition, or the precision of a recipe lies the potential for a profound sense of accomplishment and joy. This section navigates the psychological landscape of why engaging in hobbies is not just a luxury but a necessity for a well-balanced life.

Consider the concept of 'flow'—that magical state where time seems to stand still, and you are completely immersed in the activity at hand. Hobbies, when pursued with passion, have the enchanting ability to induce this state of flow, offering a respite from the ceaseless demands of the professional world. The joy derived from a hobby is not just a fleeting moment of happiness; it's a sustainable wellspring of positive emotions that nourishes the soul.

Moreover, there's a profound role that hobbies play in shaping one's identity. In a world often defined by job titles and professional achievements, engaging in hobbies becomes a declaration of individuality. Whether you're a weekend gardener, an amateur astronomer, or a fervent reader, your hobbies contribute to the mosaic of your identity—a reminder that you are more than the sum of your professional endeavors.

Balancing Hobbies with Work and Family

In the intricate dance of work-life balance, one of the key challenges is the seamless integration of hobbies into a schedule dominated by professional commitments and familial responsibilities. This part of the chapter unravels the delicate art of balancing passions with the demands of the outside world.

Time, a currency often scarce in the professional realm, becomes a central focus. The chapter delves into the concept of time management, urging individuals to view the time allocated for hobbies not as an indulgence but as an essential investment in well-being. It's about recognizing the importance of carving out dedicated moments for activities that bring joy and fulfillment.

Boundaries emerge as stalwart guardians of these precious pockets of hobby time. Just as boundaries are vital in the professional arena, they play an equally crucial role in safeguarding the sanctity of personal pursuits. Communicating these boundaries becomes a form of self-advocacy—a declaration that personal passions deserve a space untouched by the encroachments of work or family obligations.

Furthermore, the chapter recognizes the dynamic nature of balance, understanding that there will be seasons where professional demands take precedence and others where personal passions become the guiding stars. It's not about a rigid equilibrium but a fluid adaptation to the ever-shifting currents of life—a recognition that the pursuit of balance is a journey, not a destination.

Chapter Fourteen

Lifelong Learning and Continued Professional Development

In the dynamic landscape of the modern professional world, the concept of education transcends the traditional boundaries of classrooms and degrees. Lifelong learning and continued professional development have emerged as not just buzzwords but as indispensable strategies for success. In this chapter, we embark on a journey through the realms of continuous learning, exploring the why, the how, and the myriad benefits it brings to the professional journey.

In the not-so-distant past, education was often viewed as a finite endeavor—a phase of life dedicated to acquiring knowledge and skills that would set the foundation for a career. However, the rapid pace of technological advancement, the globalization of industries, and the ever-shifting demands of the job market have rendered the traditional model of education insufficient.

Lifelong learning is not a luxury reserved for the intellectually curious; it's a strategic imperative for the modern professional. The skills and knowledge that were cutting-edge yesterday might be obsolete tomorrow. As industries evolve and job roles transform, the ability to adapt and learn becomes a defining factor in professional resilience.

The narrative of lifelong learning is not confined to acquiring additional degrees; it's a mindset that values continuous improvement, embraces curiosity, and sees challenges as opportunities for growth. Whether you're a seasoned executive or an entry-level professional, the commitment to lifelong learning positions you as an agile contributor to your field.

Continuous Professional Development (CPD) is the deliberate and conscious effort to enhance professional knowledge, skills, and competencies throughout one's career. It's a proactive approach to staying relevant, competitive, and proficient in a rapidly changing professional landscape.

One of the key drivers of CPD is the recognition that learning is not a one-time event but a process woven into the fabric of daily professional life. It's not about cramming information for an exam but about cultivating a habit of curiosity and a willingness to acquire new skills organically. CPD is the acknowledgment that, in the age of information, the ability to learn and unlearn is as critical as the knowledge itself.

The Four Pillars of Lifelong Learning and CPD

Technical Proficiency:

Lifelong learning in the professional sphere often begins with a commitment to technical proficiency. In fields where advancements are a constant, staying abreast of the latest technologies, methodologies, and industry trends is non-negotiable. This pillar of learning involves attending workshops, webinars, and conferences, pursuing online courses, and engaging in hands-on projects that challenge and expand your technical skill set.

Soft Skills Enhancement

While technical proficiency is a cornerstone, the modern professional landscape places equal emphasis on soft skills—those intangible qualities that define effective communication, leadership, and collaboration. Lifelong learning in this realm involves honing skills such as emotional intelligence, communication, adaptability, and leadership. It's about understanding the nuances of human interaction and developing the interpersonal skills that transcend roles and industries.

Industry and Market Insight

Lifelong learners recognize the importance of understanding the broader context in which they operate. This involves staying informed about industry trends, market dynamics, and global developments that might impact their profession. Subscribing to industry publications, participating in forums and discussion groups, and seeking mentorship from seasoned professionals are all avenues through which one can gain valuable insights beyond the confines of their immediate job responsibilities.

Personal and Professional Well-being

The holistic professional understands that learning extends beyond the confines of a job description. It encompasses personal development, well-being, and a balanced approach to life. Lifelong learners invest time in activities that promote mental and physical health, recognizing that a healthy, fulfilled individual is better equipped to navigate the challenges of a demanding professional life.

The Benefits of Lifelong Learning and CPD

The decision to embrace lifelong learning and continuous professional development is not just an investment in one's career; it's a commitment to personal and intellectual growth. Here are some of the myriad benefits that this commitment brings:

Adaptability in a Changing Landscape

The professional landscape is akin to a constantly evolving ecosystem. Lifelong learners are equipped with the adaptability needed to thrive in this dynamic environment. They don't see change as a threat but as an invitation to learn, grow, and contribute in new and innovative ways.

Enhanced Problem-Solving Skills

Lifelong learning is, at its core, about developing a problem-solving mindset. The ability to approach challenges with a curious, solution-oriented perspective is a hallmark of those committed to continuous improvement. Lifelong learners are not daunted by obstacles; they view them as opportunities to apply and expand their knowledge and skills.

Career Resilience

The job market is no longer a static landscape. Lifelong learners are resilient in the face of economic uncertainties, industry shifts, and technological disruptions. Their commitment to staying current and relevant positions them as assets in times of change rather than liabilities.

Professional Satisfaction and Fulfillment

Lifelong learning is not a burdensome obligation but a source of professional satisfaction. The joy of acquiring new skills, the fulfillment of overcoming challenges, and the intellectual stimulation that comes with continuous learning contribute to a sense of purpose and engagement in one's professional journey.

Leadership Development

The most effective leaders are often the most avid learners. Lifelong learning is a cornerstone of leadership development. Whether you're leading a team or steering an organization, the ability to inspire, communicate effectively, and navigate complex challenges requires a commitment to ongoing self-improvement.

Importance of Continuous Learning

In the ever-evolving tapestry of the professional world, the significance of continuous learning stands as a beacon guiding individuals through the dynamic landscape. This section will delve into the multifaceted importance of embracing a commitment to lifelong learning and its profound impact on professional adaptability, skill enhancement, and personal fulfillment.

Continuous learning is the linchpin in the dynamic professional landscape. In a world where change is constant, adapting is not just a survival strategy—it's a pathway to success. This part uncovers the symbiotic dance between continuous learning and adaptability. We'll explore how staying ahead in terms of industry shifts, technological advancements, and global trends positions individuals not just as survivors but as architects of change.

Take the IT industry, for instance. Professionals who made continuous learning a habit found themselves at the forefront of emerging technologies. They didn't just adapt; they shaped the narrative. We'll journey through stories of professionals who turned challenges into stepping stones by embracing a commitment to continuous learning.

Continuous learning isn't just about staying current; it's about expanding your toolkit. This section will unravel how skill enhancement through continuous learning opens doors to new opportunities. Think of it like a craftsman adding new tools to their kit. We'll explore case studies of individuals who, through strategic skill enhancement, seamlessly transitioned between roles, tackled diverse challenges, and emerged as versatile assets in a competitive job market.

It's not just technical skills; it's about soft skills too. Effective communication, emotional intelligence, and leadership are as crucial as technical proficiency. Continuous learning becomes a holistic journey that hones both the hard and soft facets of professional prowess.

Beyond the career perks, continuous learning weaves a tapestry of personal fulfillment and intellectual growth. Let's dive into the intrinsic rewards of a commitment to lifelong learning. We'll explore how the pursuit of knowledge becomes a journey of self-discovery, curiosity, and intellectual stimulation.

Continuous learners aren't just ticking off boxes for external validation; they find joy in the process of learning itself. This joy transcends the confines of a job description or career aspirations—it becomes a source of intrinsic motivation that fuels a lifelong quest for knowledge. Through anecdotes and insights, we'll delve into the transformative power of continuous learning in fostering a sense of purpose, engagement, and intellectual fulfillment.

Adapting to the Ever-Changing Professional Landscape

In an era where change is the only constant, professionals must equip themselves with the tools necessary to navigate the twists and turns of the ever-changing landscape. Continuous learning emerges as the compass that not only points the way forward but also empowers individuals to thrive amidst uncertainty. This segment will explore the symbiotic relationship between continuous learning and adaptability, emphasizing the role of knowledge acquisition in staying ahead of industry shifts, technological advancements, and global trends.

As industries undergo rapid transformations, those who embrace continuous learning emerge as architects of change rather than casualties. The ability to adapt isn't merely a survival skill; it's a strategic advantage that positions individuals as invaluable contributors in a world where stagnation is the precursor to obsolescence. We'll delve into real-world examples of professionals who, through a commitment to continuous learning, have not only weathered storms of change but have also emerged as leaders shaping the direction of their industries.

Enhancing Skill Sets for Future Opportunities

Continuous learning is the alchemy that transforms professionals into perpetual learners, forever expanding their arsenal of skills and competencies. This section will unravel the symbiotic relationship between skill enhancement and future opportunities, exploring how a proactive approach to learning opens doors to new roles, responsibilities, and career trajectories.

The modern professional is akin to a craftsman refining their tools, recognizing that each new skill acquired is not just a feather in their cap but a key that unlocks doors to uncharted territories. We'll explore case studies of individuals who, through strategic skill enhancement, have transitioned seamlessly between roles, tackled diverse challenges, and positioned themselves as versatile assets in a competitive job market.

Furthermore, the discussion will extend beyond technical skills to encompass the vital realm of soft skills. In a landscape where effective communication, emotional intelligence, and leadership are as crucial as technical proficiency, continuous learning becomes a holistic journey that hones both the hard and soft facets of professional prowess.

Personal Fulfillment and Intellectual Growth

Beyond the pragmatic advantages, continuous learning weaves a tapestry of personal fulfillment and intellectual growth. This segment will unravel the intrinsic rewards of a commitment to lifelong learning, exploring how the pursuit of knowledge becomes a journey of self-discovery, curiosity, and intellectual stimulation.

Continuous learners aren't driven solely by external motivations; they find joy in the process of learning itself. This joy transcends the confines of a job description or career aspirations—it becomes a source of intrinsic motivation that fuels a lifelong quest for knowledge. Through anecdotes and insights, we'll delve into the transformative power of continuous learning in fostering a sense of purpose, engagement, and intellectual fulfillment.

The discussion will extend to the concept of intellectual growth as a dynamic and ongoing process. Continuous learners understand that the mind, like a muscle, thrives on regular exercise. We'll explore how embracing challenges, pursuing new interests, and constantly pushing intellectual boundaries contribute not only to professional success but also to a richer, more meaningful life.

Utilizing Online Resources and Platforms

In the digital era, the avenues for continuous learning have expanded exponentially, with online resources and platforms emerging as the cornerstone of professional development. This section delves into the practical aspects of leveraging online resources, exploring popular platforms for professional courses, the delicate balance between quality and cost, and strategies for staying abreast of ever-evolving industry trends.

Popular Platforms for Professional Courses

The digital realm teems with platforms offering a smorgasbord of professional courses, each vying for attention and promising to be the gateway to skill enhancement and career advancement. One such behemoth in the online learning landscape is LinkedIn Learning. Renowned for its extensive library of courses spanning a myriad of industries, LinkedIn Learning provides a platform for professionals to acquire both technical and soft skills.

Coursera, a trailblazer in the realm of Massive Open Online Courses (MOOCs), partners with universities and organizations to deliver courses ranging from data science to leadership skills. Its interactive and collaborative approach to learning has garnered a global following.

For those seeking technical proficiency, Udacity focuses on courses in programming, data science, and artificial intelligence. Known for its nano degree programs, Udacity tailors its content to industry needs, providing learners with hands-on projects and real-world applications.

The list extends to platforms like edX, Skillshare, and Pluralsight, each with its unique offerings and strengths. EdX, a nonprofit founded by Harvard and MIT, boasts a diverse range of courses from top universities. Skillshare, on the other hand, thrives on a model of creativity and collaboration, with courses spanning design, writing, and entrepreneurship. Pluralsight zeroes in on technology-related courses, making it a go-to for IT professionals seeking to stay ahead in a rapidly evolving landscape.

The discussion will not only highlight the variety of platforms available but also guide readers in choosing the one that aligns with their learning style, career goals, and budget constraints.

Balancing Quality with Cost

While the accessibility of online courses is unparalleled, the age-old adage "you get what you pay for" echoes through the virtual halls of digital learning. This section addresses the delicate dance of balancing quality with cost, offering insights into how professionals can maximize the value of their investment in online courses.

Free courses abound on platforms like Khan Academy and Codecademy, providing a gateway for those on a tight budget. However, the trade-off often lies in the depth and specificity of the content. Aspiring professionals can dip their toes into various subjects, but for a comprehensive mastery, a more substantial investment may be necessary.

Paid platforms such as LinkedIn Learning and Coursera come with a price tag, yet they offer a trove of high-quality content. The discussion will delve into strategies for making informed choices, including reading reviews, exploring free trials, and considering the reputation of the instructors and institutions behind the courses.

Moreover, the conversation extends beyond the initial cost to the long-term value of the investment. A course might be expensive, but if it catalyzes a career advancement or a significant skill upgrade, the return on investment becomes evident. The focus will be on empowering professionals to view online courses not just as expenses but as strategic investments in their continuous learning journey.

Staying Updated with Industry Trends

The professional landscape is a dynamic tapestry of evolving trends, and staying ahead requires a keen awareness of industry shifts. Online learning platforms can serve as not just repositories of knowledge but as dynamic channels for staying updated with the latest trends.

Platforms like LinkedIn Learning often collaborate with industry experts to deliver courses that align with current trends. These platforms leverage their vast user base to identify emerging skills and technologies, ensuring that professionals have access to timely and relevant content.

Beyond formal courses, online communities and forums play a pivotal role in staying abreast of industry trends. Reddit, Stack Overflow, and industry-specific forums serve as virtual watercoolers where professionals exchange insights, discuss emerging technologies, and share experiences. The section will guide professionals on how to leverage these online communities effectively, transforming them into valuable sources of industry intelligence.

The conversation will also touch upon the importance of cultivating a personal learning network. Following thought leaders on platforms like Twitter and subscribing to industry newsletters can provide a steady stream of curated content and insights. Professionals will be encouraged to embrace a proactive approach to staying updated, recognizing that continuous learning extends beyond the confines of formal courses.

Attending Workshops, Seminars, and Conferences

The allure of live events—workshops, seminars, and conferences—is embedded in the tangible energy of shared knowledge, the buzz of networking opportunities, and the immersion in a collective pursuit of professional excellence. In this section, we will unravel the multifaceted advantages of attending such events, exploring the realms of networking, staying updated with industry best practices, and the practical implementation of newfound knowledge in day-to-day work.

Networking Opportunities and Peer Learning

Live events serve as dynamic ecosystems where professionals from diverse backgrounds converge, creating fertile ground for networking opportunities and peer learning. The bustling corridors of a conference or the interactive sessions of a workshop become more than physical spaces; they transform into arenas for the exchange of ideas, and experiences, and the forging of professional connections.

This section will delve into the art of networking, offering insights into how professionals can navigate these events strategically. From approaching keynote speakers to engaging in meaningful conversations during networking breaks, we'll explore practical tips for building a network that transcends the boundaries of the event itself.

Moreover, the discussion will extend to the power of peer learning—the invaluable insights gained from fellow professionals facing similar challenges. Workshops and seminars, often designed as interactive forums, provide opportunities for collaborative problem-solving and the exchange of best practices. Real-world examples will illustrate how professionals, through active participation in these events, have not only expanded their knowledge base but have also formed lasting professional alliances.

Staying Updated with Industry Best Practices

The professional landscape is a dynamic tapestry of evolving best practices, and attending live events becomes a conduit for staying at the forefront of industry trends. Whether it's a seminar on the latest advancements in technology or a workshop on innovative management strategies, live events offer a real-time pulse of industry best practices.

This section will guide professionals on how to navigate the diverse offerings of these events to stay updated strategically. From selecting sessions that align with current industry challenges to engaging with exhibitors showcasing cutting-edge solutions, professionals will gain insights into maximizing the impact of their event attendance.

Furthermore, the discussion will highlight the role of thought leaders and industry experts who often grace these events as keynote speakers. Their presentations offer a glimpse into emerging trends, future projections, and the evolving landscape of best practices. Attendees will be encouraged to not only absorb this information but to actively engage in Q&A sessions and discussions to deepen their understanding.

Implementing Learnings in Day-to-Day Work

The true litmus test of any learning experience lies in its practical application. This section will explore strategies for professionals to seamlessly integrate the knowledge gained from workshops, seminars, and conferences into their day-to-day work.

One key aspect is note-taking and reflection during the event itself. Professionals will be encouraged to adopt effective note-taking practices, capturing not just facts but personal insights and action points. These notes become valuable reference material when translating theoretical knowledge into actionable strategies in the workplace.

The role of post-event reflection will also be emphasized. Taking the time to digest information, identify key takeaways, and create an actionable plan ensures that the investment in attending the event translates into tangible outcomes. Case studies will illustrate how professionals have successfully implemented learnings, resulting in enhanced efficiency, innovative problem-solving, and, ultimately, career advancement.

Moreover, the section will address the importance of sharing insights with colleagues who may not have attended the event. Creating a culture of knowledge sharing within the workplace ensures that the benefits of attending live events permeate the entire team, contributing to a collective elevation of skills and performance.

Seeking Feedback and Peer Reviews

In the pursuit of continuous learning and professional growth, seeking feedback and embracing peer reviews emerge as indispensable tools. Feedback, when sought earnestly, acts as a mirror reflecting not just our strengths but also the areas where growth is possible. It's a compass guiding us toward refinement and evolution. Embracing feedback requires humility and a genuine desire to elevate one's performance.

Peer reviews, in particular, harness the collective intelligence of a team or community. They provide a panoramic view of our contributions, offering diverse perspectives and insights. Beyond the constructive criticism lies the invaluable gem of affirmation—an acknowledgment of the strengths we bring to the table.

Moreover, the art of seeking feedback is reciprocal. By inviting others to share their perspectives, we create a culture of openness and collaboration. It's a symbiotic exchange where everyone becomes a catalyst for each other's professional development.

Constructive Criticism as a Growth Tool

The concept of constructive criticism often dances on the fine line between discomfort and growth. However, understanding and embracing this tool is fundamental to the journey of continuous improvement. Constructive criticism is not a mere pointing out of flaws; it's a strategic unveiling of areas for enhancement coupled with actionable insights for development.

In the professional sphere, where the stakes are high and the pursuit of excellence is relentless, constructive criticism becomes the compass guiding individuals toward mastery. This part will explore the psychological nuances of receiving constructive criticism, emphasizing the importance of cultivating a growth mindset.

The focus will shift to viewing constructive criticism not as a threat but as an invaluable resource for refinement. Professionals will be encouraged to reframe their perspective, recognizing that feedback is not a judgment but an opportunity—an opportunity to refine skills, improve performance, and ultimately, to excel in their chosen field.

Regularly Scheduling Feedback Sessions

Feedback is not a sporadic event but a continuous process embedded in the fabric of professional development. This section will elucidate the importance of scheduling regular feedback sessions, whether they are formal evaluations with supervisors or informal discussions with peers.

Formal feedback sessions with supervisors are often built into the annual performance review structure of organizations. However, this section will advocate for a more proactive approach, encouraging professionals to seek feedback beyond the prescribed timelines. The conversation will extend to the art of initiating these discussions, ensuring they are constructive dialogues rather than stressful interrogations.

Informal feedback sessions with peers will also be explored as a valuable avenue for growth. Peer reviews provide a unique perspective, often offering insights that might not be apparent to a supervisor. Professionals will be guided on how to navigate these conversations, fostering an environment of mutual respect and constructive exchange.

The key takeaway will be the integration of feedback sessions into the routine of professional life. Rather than viewing them as occasional check-ins, professionals will be empowered to see feedback as a consistent and vital element of their journey toward excellence.

Turning Feedback into Actionable Steps

Feedback, when treated as a checklist of suggestions, often falls short of its transformative potential. This section will illuminate the strategic art of turning feedback into actionable steps. It's not merely about acknowledging areas for improvement; it's about crafting a roadmap for growth.

Professionals will be guided through the process of dissecting feedback, identifying recurring themes, and distilling actionable insights. The conversation will delve into the importance of setting specific, measurable, achievable, relevant, and time-bound (SMART) goals based on the feedback received.

Moreover, this part will explore the significance of accountability in the feedback loop. It's not just about receiving feedback; it's about taking ownership of the development journey. Professionals will be encouraged to view feedback as a partnership between themselves and their growth aspirations, recognizing that the onus is on them to translate insights into action.

Real-world examples of individuals who have leveraged feedback as a catalyst for significant growth will be interwoven into the narrative. These stories will serve as beacons, illustrating how actionable steps, when fueled by constructive criticism, can propel professionals toward unprecedented heights in their careers.

Chapter Fifteen

The Role of Certifications and Advanced Degrees

In the ever-evolving landscape of professional development, the pursuit of certifications and advanced degrees stands as a pivotal avenue for career enhancement. This section delves into the multifaceted role of certifications and advanced degrees, examining the dynamics of return on investment, strategies for staying updated with relevant certifications, and the delicate art of balancing education with work commitments.

Analyzing the Return on Investment for Advanced Education

Investing time and resources in advanced education is akin to planting seeds with the expectation of a bountiful harvest. This segment explores the nuances of return on investment (ROI) for advanced degrees, shedding light on how professionals can assess and maximize the value of their educational pursuits.

While the allure of an advanced degree is often tied to the promise of career advancement and increased earning potential, the discussion will extend beyond the immediate benefits. Professionals will be guided in analyzing how an advanced degree aligns with their long-term career goals, the trajectory of their industry, and the evolving demands of the job market.

Case studies of individuals who strategically navigated advanced education to catapult their careers will be explored. The emphasis will be on understanding that ROI extends beyond financial gains—it encompasses the acquisition of in-depth knowledge, expanded networks, and the cultivation of critical thinking skills that transcend the boundaries of a specific role.

Additionally, the section will address the evolving landscape of remote and online education, providing insights into how professionals can leverage virtual learning environments for advanced degrees. It will explore the benefits and potential pitfalls of online education, equipping readers with the tools to make informed decisions about the format and structure of their advanced education.

Staying Updated with Relevant Certifications

In a world where the half-life of skills is shrinking, certifications emerge as badges of currency, tangible proof of a professional's commitment to staying relevant in their field. This part will dissect the strategic role of certifications, offering insights into how professionals can navigate the labyrinth of options and choose certifications that align with their career aspirations.

Certifications, whether in IT, project management, or specialized fields, serve as micro-credentials attesting to a professional's proficiency in a specific domain. The discussion will explore how the right certifications can open doors to new opportunities, differentiate professionals in a competitive job market, and serve as a continuous validation of their expertise.

Furthermore, the section will guide professionals in staying updated with relevant certifications, considering the rapid evolution of industries and technologies. Strategies for identifying emerging certifications, understanding their value in the job market, and incorporating them into a continuous learning plan will be unpacked.

Case studies will illuminate professionals who strategically navigated the certification landscape, showcasing how these credentials became catalysts for career growth. The emphasis will be on approaching certifications not as isolated achievements but as building blocks in a comprehensive strategy for continuous professional development.

Balancing Education with Work

The pursuit of advanced degrees and certifications often unfolds against the backdrop of a demanding professional life. This section will delve into the art of balancing education with work commitments, offering practical strategies for professionals juggling the dual responsibilities of career advancement and ongoing learning.

Time management becomes a linchpin in this delicate balancing act. The discussion will explore techniques for effective time management, including creating dedicated study schedules, leveraging breaks and downtime, and prioritizing tasks based on urgency and importance.

Moreover, professionals will be encouraged to foster open communication with employers and supervisors regarding their educational pursuits. Strategies for articulating the benefits of ongoing education to employers, seeking support for flexible work arrangements, and aligning educational goals with organizational objectives will be explored.

The section will also address the evolving landscape of remote work, providing insights into how professionals can seamlessly integrate education into their work-from-home routines. It will explore the benefits of virtual learning environments, online collaboration tools, and the flexibility they afford to those seeking to balance education with professional commitments.

Chapter Sixteen

Conclusion

After an enlightening journey through the intricacies of professional confidence, it's clear that navigating the corporate landscape is an ongoing process. The evolution of corporate culture, explored in the initial chapters, underscores the importance of aligning personal values with the dynamic expectations of the modern workplace. As we transition from the traditional corporate ladder to flexible structures, the emphasis on soft skills, emotional intelligence, and the impact of technology becomes evident.

Mastering interpersonal relationships, as highlighted in Chapter 2, emerges as a cornerstone. Building trust, effective communication, and understanding office politics are vital skills. Empathy and emotional intelligence, often overlooked, are key ingredients in successful professional relationships.

The exploration of leadership in Chapter 3 extends beyond titles. Inclusive leadership, effective decision-making, and leading during crises are crucial aspects. The emphasis on continuous learning and adaptability is a reminder that leadership is a journey, not a destination.

"Branding Yourself" is not just a buzzword; it's about understanding and consistently projecting your professional identity. Managing your digital footprint, networking strategically, and embracing thought leadership contribute to a robust personal brand. The importance of feedback in this process cannot be overstated.

The chapter on job interviews is a practical guide, emphasizing the significance of preparation, non-verbal communication, and follow-up strategies. Success in interviews is not just about showcasing skills but demonstrating cultural fit and soft skills.

Navigating career changes and transitions, discussed in Chapter 6, requires recognizing when change is necessary, strategizing the next move, and managing the emotional rollercoaster. The importance of a structured onboarding process in a new role cannot be overlooked.

Chapter 7 delves into achieving work-life balance, challenging the myth of "having it all." Setting boundaries, effective time management, stress management, and pursuing hobbies are integral to a satisfying and balanced life.

The final chapter, focusing on lifelong learning and continued professional development, underscores the importance of adapting to change. Utilizing online resources, attending workshops, seeking feedback, and balancing education with work contribute to sustained growth.

In conclusion, professional confidence is not a destination but a continuous journey. This book serves as a guide through the evolving landscape of corporate culture, interpersonal relationships, leadership, personal branding, interviews, career changes, work-life balance, and lifelong learning. The key takeaway is the encouragement to take proactive steps and own one's career. Embrace change, cultivate relationships, and prioritize continuous learning to thrive in the dynamic world of work. As Mahatma Gandhi said, "Live as if you were to die tomorrow. Learn as if you were to live forever."

www.ingramcontent.com/pod-product-compliance
Lightning Source LLC
LaVergne TN
LVHW021824060526
838201LV00058B/3503